Women, Gender, and Health
Susan L. Smith and Nancy Tomes, Series Editors

# Nursing and the Privilege of Prescription, 1893–2000

Arlene W. Keeling

The Ohio State University Press
Columbus

Cataloging-in-Publication Data
Keeling, Arlene W., 1948–
      Nursing and the privilege of prescription, 1893–2000 / Arlene W.
Keeling.
            p. ; cm. — (Women, gender, and health)
      Includes bibliographical references and index.
      ISBN-13: 978-0-8142-1050-5 (cloth : alk. paper)
      ISBN-10: 0-8142-1050-3 (cloth : alk. paper)
      1. Nursing—United States—History—20th century.  2. Drugs—
Prescribing—United States—History—20th century.   I. Title. II. Series.
      [DNLM: 1. Nursing Services—history—United States.  2. History,
19th Century—United States.  3. History, 20th Century—United States.
      4. Nurse's Role—history—United States.  5. Prescriptions, Drug—
history—United States.    WY 11 AA1 K26n 2007]
      RT31.K444 2007
      610.73—dc22

                                                          2006025073

Cover design by Jay Bastian
Type set in Adobe Garamond
Printed by Thomson-Shore, Inc.

9 8 7 6 5 4 3 2 1

*This book is dedicated to my mother, Charlotte Elizabeth Prins Wynbeek, who introduced me to the world of the library and instilled in me a love of women's history. It is also dedicated to the nurses and physicians whose story is told within these pages.*

# CONTENTS

# List of Illustrations

# List of Abbreviations

| | |
|---|---|
| AANA HF | American Association of Nurse Anesthetists, Historical Files |
| *AJN* | *American Journal of Nursing* |
| *AJS, JA* | *American Journal of Surgery, Anesthesia Supplement* |
| *BHM* | *Bulletin of the History of Medicine* |
| BIA | Bureau of Indian Affairs |
| CNHI, UVA | Center for Nursing Historical Inquiry, The University of Virginia |
| CSHN, UP | Center for the Study of the History of Nursing, The University of Pennsylvania |
| CU | Columbia University |
| FNS Routine | Frontier Nursing Service Medical Routines (standing orders) |
| FNSC, UK-SC | Frontier Nursing Service Collection, University of Kentucky, Division of Special Collections & Archives |
| IHS | Indian Health Service |
| IHSNQ | Indian Health Service Nursing Questionnaires |
| *JAANA* | *Journal of the American Association of Nurse Anesthetists* |
| *JAMA* | *Journal of the American Medical Association* |
| KC-CNHI | Keeling Collection, Center for Nursing Historical Inquiry |
| KHSLSC-UL | Kornhsuser Health Sciences Library Special Collections, University of Louisville |
| LWC | Lillian Ward Collection |
| MCC | Mary Clymer Collection |
| NARA | National Archives Records Administration, Washington, DC |
| NAU-BBWC | Northern Arizona University—Virginia Brown, Ida Bahl & Lillian Watson Collection |
| NAU-CL | Northern Arizona University, Cline Library Special Collections & Archives Department |
| *NHR* | *Nursing History Review* |
| NYPL | New York Public Library |
| PC, CNHI | Pinneo Collection, Center for Nursing Historical Inquiry |
| PCH, CNHI | Peach Collection, Center for Nursing Historical Inquiry |
| *PHQ* | *Public Health Quarterly* |

| | |
|---|---|
| *QSAA, AJS* | *Quarterly Supplement of Anesthesia & Analgesia, American Journal of Surgery* |
| RWJ | Robert Wood Johnson Foundation |
| *SLLJ* | *St. Louis Law Journal* |
| USPHS | United States Public Health Service |
| VCU | Virginia Commonwealth University |
| WPA | Works Progress Administration |

# Acknowledgments

This book could not have been written without financial support from the National Library of Medicine at the National Institute of Health (G13–LM07604–02) and the National Institute of Nursing Research (K01) and the help and support of friends, colleagues, and archivists across the nation, and for all of this assistance I am grateful. First and foremost, I am indebted to Barbara Brodie for introducing me to the study of nursing history early in my graduate career and for mentoring me along this incredible journey, and to Joan Lynaugh for her mentorship, friendship, support, and insightful critique of the work. Joan also gave me permission to use her words "necessary knowledge for safe care" as a unifying theme, and for that I express my gratitude. A special thanks also goes to Julie Fairman, Pat D'Antonio, and Karen Buhler Wilkerson for their insightful questions and comments about the research and my conclusions, and to the nurses and physicians I interviewed on the telephone or in person, including Judith Stuart, Barbara Dunn, Denise Geolot, Richard Crampton, Rose Pinneo, Janet Younger, and others too numerous to mention.

I am also indebted to the many graduate students who assisted me in data collection, including Kathleen Haugh and Nancy Jallo, who traveled with me to the "hoot owl hollers" in Kentucky; law student Erin Segal Whaley and her advisor Paul Lombardo for interpreting the legal cases for me; and John Kirchgessner, Joy Buck, Jennifer Casavant, and Gina Alexander for their endless copying of research articles and help in the archives. A special thanks also goes to colleagues who heard and reacted to early drafts of the work presented at the American Association for the History of Nursing, the Southern Association for the History of Medicine, and the American Association for the History of Medicine conferences, and to the history graduate students at the both the University of Virginia and the University of Pennsylvania whose critique also helped shape the work. In addition, this book reflects the invaluable comments from the editors and anonymous reviewers at The Ohio State University Press, and to them I am grateful.

I'd also like to thank the acute care nurse practitioner and clinical nurse specialist graduate students at the University of Virginia, and ACNP faculty Suzanne Burns, Audrey Snyder, and Nita Reigle, who kept me grounded in the realities of clinical practice while I pursued this project. I extend a special thank you to my friends, Connie and Donald Brown, and colleagues, Cheryl Bourguignon, Ann Hamric, Mary and Robert Gibson, Ann Taylor, Sharon Utz, Doris Greiner, Tina Brashers, Barbara Parker, Beth Merwin, Courtney Lyder, Pamela Kulbok, Doris Glick, JoAnne Peach, Giny Lee, Linda Davies, Dorothy Tullmann, and Rick Steeves for their support and friendship during the process. My administrative assistants Renee Breeden and Linda Hanson also deserve credit for their patience and support with the details of this project.

A special thanks also goes to my family: to my daughter Amy, who traveled with me in the summer monsoon season to the Navajo Reservation and the Cline library to collect data; to Jennifer and D'Arcy II, for getting me out of the house to see D'Arcy III—at least at dinner time; to Jennifer also for introducing me to the world of photography and the work of artists like Laura Gilpin; to my son, David, for his critique of the work through a poet's eyes, and my daughter-in-law, Jen for believing that I could do this; to Rich and Eric, for their support and a second home in New York City when I was researching the Henry Street Settlement; and to Ashby, my golden retriever, who faithfully nudged my hands off the computer so that we could take a walk.

A special thanks also goes to the archivists at the University of Virginia Health Sciences Special Collections; the Cline Library at Northern Arizona University; The New York Public Library; Columbia University; The University of Kentucky, Special Collections; The Ekstrom Library in Louisville, Kentucky; and the archives of the American Association of Nurse Anesthetists in Chicago.

Finally, I'd like to thank my sister Carol and her husband, Paul, for providing me vacations at their home in Bonita Springs, and my sister Doris Rikkers, who left her own family (thank you, Bill!) for a month in October 2005 to spend time with me at a little house on Long Beach Island where this work came to fruition. Without Doris's editing skills, support, critique, and encouragement, the book would not have been possible.

# Introduction

In January and February 2000, I received numerous e-mails on the subject of new legislation being proposed in the Virginia legislature related to expanding prescriptive authority for nurse practitioners. As director of the Acute Care Nurse Practitioner (ACNP) program at the University of Virginia, I was very interested in the issue. That year, in the Commonwealth of Virginia, nurse-practitioners were restricted to prescribing only one of six categories of drugs (legend drugs), and many of the recent graduates of our program were writing to me about the difficulties the restrictions were causing in their daily practice.

Shortly after receiving the e-mails, I expressed my interest, concern, and hope for change to a colleague in a hallway conversation. The colleague happened to be Ann B. Hamric, PhD, RN, FAAN, who had edited several books on advanced practice nursing and had presented her research data on the safety and efficacy of nurse practitioners' prescriptive practices in Louisiana to the Louisiana state legislature in 1997.[1] Ann's response was prompt: "Are you going to Richmond to testify on the nurses' behalf?" I thought for a moment and then replied: "I can't. I don't know the whole story. Nurses have been giving medicines—with or without prescriptive authority—for over a century. How can I know where we should go with all this if I don't know where we've been?" Ann's reply was direct: "Well, if you don't know and you're a nurse historian, then I don't know who does. You'd better find out."

So I wrote a grant proposal, and in 2002 the National Library of Medicine awarded me funding to research the "History of Prescriptive Authority in Nursing in the Twentieth Century" (G13). This book is the result of that three-year project and another three-year grant (K01) on the "History of Coronary Care Nursing in the United States" funded by the National Institute of Nursing Research (NINR). It is an attempt to tell the story of nurses' work with medications over the last century—a story that has the potential to shape policy decisions today in the ongoing debates about prescriptive authority for nonphysician health care providers.

The history of nurses' work with medications is, for the most part, invisible—in fact, it is absent from history books. Despite the fact that nurses administer, dispense, furnish, and/or prescribe medicines every day, the profession, as a whole, has minimized this aspect of its work, instead advertising itself as the "caring" profession and highlighting the psychosocial aspects of nurses' responsibilities. To my knowledge, with perhaps the exception of Bonnie Bullough's work *The Law and the Expanding Nursing Role*,[2] a book on this subject has not been written. Numerous articles have been published on specific aspects of prescriptive privileges for nurses, but most of those begin in 1965 with the formal development of the nurse practitioner role.

This book seeks to make visible nurses' work related to medical therapeutics. It is a short history of nursing, medicine, and prescriptive authority in the United States in the twentieth century. It is not meant to be the definitive history of twentieth-century prescriptive authority in general; nor is it simply a history of prescriptive authority for nurse anesthetists, nurse-midwives, or nurse practitioners specifically, although it is inextricably linked to those histories. Using a case study approach, the book identifies and describes the informal and formal roles nurses played over the course of the century in dispensing, furnishing, and prescribing medications. (These terms are defined as follows: [1] "to dispense" means to administer a drug from one's nursing bag or from samples; [2] "to furnish" means to give a drug according to standing orders of a physician; and [3] "to prescribe" is to write or telephone in a prescription for a specific drug to be dispensed by a pharmacist.) The book discusses the nurse's roles in the social, political, economic, and legal context in which the activities took place and in relationship to the history of nursing and medicine, while occasionally introducing the history of pharmacy (a topic which goes beyond the scope of this work). It addresses the national movement from domestic care toward scientific medical care in the early part of the century and the knowledge needed to give medical and nursing care as that care became increasingly complex.

The book is built around a series of case studies representing different geographic areas of the United States during different decades of the twentieth century. Although numerous historians have addressed specific aspects of each of the cases presented here, none has analyzed the cases through the specific lens of a history of prescriptive authority in nursing in the twentieth century. For example, much like this book does for nursing, John Warner's book, *The Therapeutic Perspective: Medical Practice, Knowledge and Identity in America, 1820–1885,* examines the relationship of therapeutic intervention and professional identity for physicians, detailing changes in therapy over time by examining physicians' work in three cities: Boston, New Orleans, and Cincinnati. And, true to its purpose, Warner's book is about the medical profession in the nineteenth century.[3] Susan Reverby's *Ordered to Care* examines the history of the nursing pro-

fession in the late nineteenth and early twentieth centuries, but that book focuses on the caring aspects of the nurse's role rather than on nursing therapeutics.[4] Rosemary Stevens masterfully documents the history of American hospitals in her book, *In Sickness and in Wealth,* focusing on "medicine, money and power," and discussing disparities in the health care system, but she clearly does not address the nurse's role within these institutions nor does she discuss the blurring of the boundaries between medicine and nursing that occurred in intensive care.[5]

Other scholars have covered the topics of each of this book's chapters in more depth, but they do not address the nurse's work specific to dispensing, furnishing, or prescribing medications and other therapies. For example, Karen Buhler-Wilkerson's *No Place like Home* provides a comprehensive account of the work of the Henry Street Settlement Visiting Nurses, but it only touches on the medication aspects of the nurse's role.[6] Nancy Tomes's article, "The Great American Medicine Show Revisited," in the *Bulletin of the History of Medicine,* provides an insightful analysis of the emergence of the modern prescription drug between 1938 and 1951, yet the article makes little mention of the nurse's role in relation to prescriptions.[7] Likewise, Barbra Mann Wall's *Unlikely Entrepreneurs* describes Catholic sisters' work in providing anesthesia during the Civil War, while Virginia Thatcher's *A History of Anesthesia* and Mariane Bankert's *Watchful Care: A History of America's Nurse Anesthetists* both provide a broad overview of the history of nurse anesthesia in the United States, but none of these works specifically analyzes the nurse anesthetist's role in relationship to prescriptive authority in nursing.[8] The same holds true for the numerous books and articles documenting the history of the Frontier Nursing Service (FNS), including Laura Ettinger's, "Nurse-Midwives, the Mass Media, and the Politics of Maternal Health Care in the United States, 1925–1955," in the *Nursing History Review,*[9] and Judith Rooks's *Midwifery and Childbirth in America.*[10] Breckenridge's own account of the FNS, *Wide Neighborhoods,* is descriptive and presents the broad picture of the inception and growth of the organization rather than focusing on the legality of the nurse's work with medications or the nurse's scope of practice.[11]

As far as nurses' work with the Bureau of Indian Affairs (BIA) is concerned, historians Emily Abel and Nancy Reifel have done a thorough job of analyzing the cultural aspects of the nurse's role in addition to describing the nursing activities in chapter 26 of Judith Leavitt's *Women and Health in America;* nonetheless, their work does not specifically address issues related to nursing's scope of practice in giving medications to the American Indians. Much the same can be said for Abel's article, "'We are left so much alone to work out our own problems': Nurses on American Indian Reservations during the 1930s," in *Nursing History Review* and

Mary Ann Ruffing-Rahal's "The Navajo Experience of Elizabeth Forster, Public Health Nurse," in another volume of the same journal. Both of these excellent articles provide a broad picture of nurses' work with the Bureau of Indian Affairs. But despite the fact that both articles reference the field nurse's use of medicines, neither specifically analyzes this aspect of the nurse's role.[12]

Related to the latter half of this book, Julie Fairman's and Joan E. Lynaugh's book, *Critical Care Nursing: A History* and Lynaugh's and Barbara L. Brush's *American Nursing: From Hospitals to Health Systems* are two of the best works analyzing the changes that occurred in nursing practice in the mid-twentieth century, yet medication administration is not their focus.[13] In her other works, Fairman's analyses in "Playing Doctor?: Nurse Practitioners, Physicians, and the Dilemma of Shared Practice," and "Watchful Vigilance: Nursing Care, Technology and the Development of Intensive Care Units,"[14] support many of my own conclusions. Of particular note, both Margarete Sandelowski's work, "The Physicians' Eyes: American Nursing and the Diagnostic Revolution in Medicine," in *Nursing History Review* and Davinia Allen's "Negotiated Boundaries" were foundational to my analysis. Numerous other works influenced my thinking related to *Nursing and the Privilege of Prescription*. These works are referenced in specific chapters.

As noted earlier, this book uses case studies to illustrate changes in nursing practice that no doubt were occurring in numerous cities, towns, and villages across the nation during the specific time periods identified. These exemplars were used intentionally to make a complicated and what could have become a lengthy and tedious history one that could be more easily read. The cases were also used to set some boundaries on the project while simultaneously providing a glimpse of nursing practice in different regions of the United States and among different ethnic groups.

The major thesis of the book is that the amount of freedom nurses have had in dispensing, furnishing, and prescribing medications has been dependent on the particular setting in which they practiced, on individual practice negotiations between physicians and nurses at the grassroots level, and on the level of trust that developed between them.[15] Even without legal prescriptive authority, nurses safely and effectively administered drugs at various times and places throughout the century. Providing care in underserved areas of the country—in urban slums, in the remote hollows of Appalachia, and on Indian reservations—nurses offered access to care to many to whom it would otherwise have been denied. Meanwhile, in operating rooms, intensive care units, and other areas of the hospital, nurses and physicians cooperated to administer care.

Dispensing drugs when necessary, furnishing drugs according to standing order sets, or de facto prescribing, nurses did what needed to be done in times and places where they were the only ones to do it, and they took responsibility for their actions. Themes that emerge are those of promoting access to care; responsibility for that care; the importance of advanced knowledge for safe practice; economic determinants of care; and interdisciplinary cooperation, collaboration, and conflict.

The struggle between organized medicine and nursing over where, to whom, and in what circumstances a practitioner is licensed to dispense, furnish, or prescribe drugs is the central tension of the book. That struggle is contrasted with what was occurring at the grassroots level, where physicians and nurses worked together on a daily basis, learning to trust each other and their respective areas of expertise.

The book then describes the "elusive and fine line" that separates nursing and medicine and the fluidity of that line.[16] When care was to be provided in remote areas of the country, in the less desirable sections of urban cities, with minority cultures, on nights and weekends, when physicians were not readily available, the boundary moved to accommodate an expanding scope of practice for nursing.

Integrating themes are the fluidity of the line separating medicine and nursing; the influence of social mores; the political and environmental setting; economics, class, race, and cultural heritage in the issue of access to health care; and the ongoing struggle to determine who decides who will govern nursing practice. Another integrating theme is that of safety in health care and who determines the amount of knowledge prerequisite for that care. These themes emerge in each chapter and can be traced throughout the book.

Chapter 1, "Midway between the Pharmacist and the Physician: The Work of the Henry Street Settlement Visiting Nurses, 1893–1944," represents nursing care provided by the Henry Street Settlement (HSS) visiting nurses in New York City in the urban Northeast at the turn of the twentieth century. From its inception in 1893 until 1944 when the social and nursing activities were separated, the Henry Street Settlement (HSS) visiting nurses linked nursing, social welfare, and the public. The HSS visiting nurses began their work on the Lower East Side of New York during the depression of 1893. Their work extended into the Progressive Era, a period in which there was a growing emphasis on widespread social and economic reform in the United States. During that time, under the rubric of social feminism, educated middle- and upper-class women like Lillian Wald and Mary Brewster participated in the movement to improve living and working conditions for poverty-stricken immigrants in the industrialized cities of the Northeast. Even in America—the land of democracy—class, race, and cultural heritage were issues.

Henry Street Settlement (HSS) Visiting Nurses provided skilled, professional nursing care to the thousands of European immigrants who crowded into ethnic ghettos in Manhattan and the surrounding areas. In addition to promoting comfort, nutrition, psychological support, and education about sanitation and health to patients and families, the HSS nurses dispensed medications from a central medicine chest located at the settlement house. In their work, the visiting nurses practiced in what Lillian Wald's close friend and colleague, Lavinia Dock, would refer to as the "middle place"—somewhere between professional medical services and unskilled family care-giving[17]—providing skilled nursing care to both middle- and working-class families, particularly to the immigrants who settled in New York City.

The Henry Street nurses practiced at the edges of their disciplinary boundaries, often diagnosing and treating commonly occurring illnesses and referring patients to physicians when necessary. In doing so, the HSS nurses worked cooperatively with local medical societies and independent physicians, but not always without interprofessional conflict. In fact, the reaction of certain divisions of the medical community that occurred in response to the HSS nurses' work was an early indication of the interprofessional conflicts that would complicate the nurse's role in relation to medications for most of the twentieth century.

Chapter 2, "Practicing Medicine without a License?: Nurse Anesthetists 1900–1938," describes and analyzes the role of nurse anesthetists during the first half of the twentieth century, particularly noting the legal complications they faced while pursuing their right to practice this specialty. In California in 1934, the Los Angeles County Medical Association, represented by William Chalmers-Francis, MD, sued nurse anesthetist Dagmar Nelson for the "illegal practice of medicine in violation of the state's medical practice act." Given the fact that nurses had been administering anesthesia since the Civil War almost seventy-five years earlier, it is interesting to speculate on how and why this lawsuit happened.

This chapter examines the history of nurse anesthesia in the United States from the late nineteenth century to 1938, identifying issues related to their scope of practice and the reaction of both organized nursing and organized medicine. During the late nineteenth and early twentieth centuries, nurses practiced the art of anesthesia unopposed—often trusted and supported by the physicians for whom they worked. However, as the practice of anesthesia became increasingly complicated and technology based, physicians began to claim ownership of the specialty. At the same time the science was advancing, World War I increased the demand for nurse anesthetists. Later, when the Great Depression created economic difficulties for physicians, further tensions would surface about the nurse anesthetist's role.

In response to each legal challenge to the nurse anesthetist's role, the Kentucky, Missouri, and California courts upheld the practice of nurse anesthesia—as long as it was the surgeon who was doing the prescribing of the anesthetic agent. These court decisions would affect the practice of nurse anesthesia for the remainder of the century. They would also influence other decisions on nursing's scope of practice. By 1938 the nursing profession had a legal precedent on which to base its tentative hold on this specialty practice. In some respects, the practice of nurse anesthesia went far beyond the boundaries of the discipline. These nurses were giving drugs that physician anesthesiologist Isabella Herb referred to as possessing "greater power for harm" than all others,[18] while other nurses working during the same period were not allowed to give an aspirin without a physician's order. Several themes emerge in this chapter: (1) specialized knowledge attained in postgraduate training programs was essential to nurse anesthetists' abilities to practice safely; (2) clinical competence in the delivery of the life-threatening anesthetic agents was prerequisite to having surgeons trust their work; and (3) publishing the results of their work enhanced nurse anesthetists' credibility.

Chapter 3, "'Providing Care in the 'Hoot Owl Hollers': Nursing, Medicine, and the Law in the Frontier Nursing Service, 1925–1950," highlights the care that the Frontier Nursing Service nurses provided to inhabitants of Leslie County, Kentucky during the early twentieth century. The chapter addresses one aspect of the Frontier Nurses' work—that of furnishing medications to patients—particularly noting the intersection of these nursing activities with medicine and the law. Two research questions are addressed: (1) how and why did the FNS obtain the support of the Kentucky medical community for their expanded role? and (2) how did the nurses' activities intersect with the federal laws regulating narcotics and the state laws regulating nursing, pharmacy, and medicine?

The answers are clear. From the late 1920s through the 1950s, nurses in the Frontier Nursing Services furnished medicines to patients in a remote, rural area of Appalachia. The time was right for the acceptance of their services on the part of the local medical community. Maternal and infant mortality in Leslie County had to be reduced.

The isolated highland region was short of physicians. There were inconsistencies in the safety and efficacy of the care provided by granny midwives, and local physicians were aware of the federal and state mandates for change. Physicians were also cognizant of the fact that the FNS nurses would not be an economic threat to them. Mary Breckenridge's Frontier Nursing Service offered a solution—one in which the physicians could take some control of obstetric care by delegating authority to educated nurse-midwives who would be under the direction of a trusted leader and friend, Mary Breckenridge.

For her part, Breckenridge was politically astute and cognizant of the law. By establishing a physician advisory committee, Breckenridge clearly acknowledged the physician's legal authority in the area of diagnosis and medical therapeutics. Rather than challenge that authority, she simply obtained physician-generated standing order sets that would enable the Frontier nurses to provide comprehensive health services in the "Hoot Owl Hollers." Practicing according to these order sets, the nurses made clinical assessments, diagnosed illnesses, and furnished medications. According to an early report by Breckenridge:

> One of the best things we have been able to do has been to effect a liaison between many of our patients and the specialists and hospitals of Lexington and Louisville. Through the kindness of the Louisville and Nashville Railroad and the generosity of the doctors, nine of whom have given their services, we were able, in the first 10 months, to give the best Kentucky has to offer to fifteen of her isolated people and this second summer several specialists have come up to hold clinics: diagnostic, gynecological and prenatal, eye, ear, nose and throat.[19]

Supported by the local medical community and the law, the Frontier nurses had unprecedented autonomy to practice nursing in an expanded role, providing holistic, culturally sensitive nursing and medical care to the people of Leslie County, Kentucky.

Chapter 4, "My Treatment Was Castor Oil and Aspirin: Field Nursing in the Indian Health Service, 1925–1955," analyzes the care provided by field nurses working with the Navajo Indians in Arizona and New Mexico from the 1930s to the 1950s. Their work under the BIA was part of a major federal government initiative to provide health care to American Indians[20] on reservations throughout the United States. There, the intersection of federal bureaucracy; meager Congressional appropriations; and professional, geographic, and environmental factors shaped the nurses' work. Bound by bureaucratic red tape and regulations, but expected to teach health promotion and disease prevention as well as transport sick patients to hospitals, visit patients at home, and care for Indian children in boarding schools, BIA nurses increased their scope of practice to do what needed to be done. They diagnosed everything from trachoma to ruptured appendices, transported critically ill patients to hospitals, taught mothers how to feed and clothe their infants, and furnished medications according to standing orders.

The BIA nurses stretched the boundaries of their professional work, making independent clinical decisions when necessary and at other times collaborating with physicians. Those nurses who were culturally sensitive and respectful of the Navajos' traditional beliefs and ceremonies for healing the sick frequently collaborated with the medicine men, as well, using their own treatments (like aspirin and cough medicine) as adjunct therapies when they were requested to do so.

Technically, the BIA nurses worked under physician supervision, but in reality the nurses often worked on their own—sometimes in telephone consultation with physicians. In their work, the field nurses made clinical decisions based on their advanced training in public health nursing and their experience in clinical practice. Clearly, much of their work stretched the traditional boundaries of nursing.

Chapter 5, "Verbal Orders and Hospital Nursing: Expanding Nurses' Scope of Practice in the Mid-Twentieth Century," addresses the changes that occurred in hospital nursing during the mid-twentieth century. Beginning with hospital nursing in the 1930s, this chapter discusses the medication nurse's responsibilities and role in administering drugs. The chapter focuses on the requirement that hospital nurses were to practice only under written physician orders. Later, with the development of intensive coronary care units, a new role for nurses emerged, and nurses expanded their scope of practice. Using cutting-edge, space-age cardiac monitoring equipment, coronary care unit (CCU) nurses interpreted cardiac arrhythmias and made clinical decisions on which they based their care. Indeed, CCU nurses shared medical knowledge with cardiologists, often surpassing the skills of general practitioners in the area of cardiac arrhythmia interpretation and management.

The chapter includes information about the creation of the Hartford CCU at Bethany Hospital in Kansas City in 1962, and the research project in the coronary care unit at Presbyterian Hospital in Philadelphia, where Dr. Lawrence E. Meltzer, Dr. J. Roderick Kitchell, and registered nurse Rose Pinneo worked collaboratively to develop a new role for nursing. In one section, called "After Midnight," the chapter explores time as place, and demonstrates how the life-saving medical treatment of cardiac defibrillation and the administration of emergency intravenous cardiac medications were rapidly delegated to nurses. Doctors shared knowledge because it made sense to do so to accomplish a greater goal, to decrease deaths from heart attacks (referred to as *myocardial infarction, or MI*) but also because it was more convenient for nurses to do more, especially at night. Viewed from either the nurse's or the physician's perspective, what the nurse could diagnose and treat "after midnight" was remarkably different from what she was responsible for during the day when the physician was present in the unit. Themes that emerge are physician-nurse cooperation and trust at a grassroots level, barriers to expanding scope of practice, and the emergence of specialty knowledge for advanced nursing practice.

Chapter 6, "Nurse Practitioners and the Prescription Pad, 1965–1980," reviews the inception and development of the idea of the pediatric nurse-practitioner in Colorado under the leadership of Loretta Ford, RN and Henry Silver, MD, and the subsequent spread of nurse-practitioner programs throughout the United States. It opens with an example of the employment of a nurse practitioner by the Indian Health Service and discusses the influence of physician shortages, particularly in rural areas, on the growth of the nurse-practitioner role. The chapter also addresses the movement toward integrating nurse-practitioner programs into master's programs in nursing. It emphasizes the importance of both public and private funding on nursing education and the growth of nurse-practitioner programs, as well as the intraprofessional and interprofessional conflict over the developing nurse-practitioner role. These issues are contrasted with the collaboration that was occurring between physicians and nurse practitioners at the grassroots level.

One section of the chapter revisits the Frontier Nursing Service and focuses on the procedures that the FNS put in place to facilitate nurse practitioners writing prescriptions in the 1970s. That section emphasizes the fact that nurse practitioners in the Frontier service were doing everything necessary to prescribe a medication except signing the prescription. (Of note, nurse midwives, introduced in chapter 3 in the Frontier Nursing Service, are dropped from follow-up because their requirements for educational preparation and certification have been outside mainstream nursing.)

Chapter 7, "Prescriptive Authority for Advanced Practice Nurses, 1980–2000," traces selected nurse practitioner and nurse anesthetist developments through the 1980s and 1990s, highlighting important legislation and issues related to the distribution of medications, and including an example of how nurse practitioners gained the right to prescribe in the Commonwealth of Virginia in 2000. The chapter opens with an e-mail I received in February 2000 about what was occurring in the Virginia state legislature regarding nurses and prescriptive authority. The chapter then reviews the scheduling of drugs by the federal government, the challenge to nurse practitioner practice that occurred in Missouri in the 1980s, the Nursing Diagnosis movement, American Medical Association (AMA) opposition in 1984, and nurse practitioners' gradual success in changing state nurse practice acts. Also included in this chapter are brief overviews of the rise of acute care nurse practitioners (ACNPs), a discussion of the implications of managed care on nursing and medical practice in the 1990s, law professor Barbara Safriet's commentary on the issues, and a challenge to nurse practitioner practice published in the *New England Journal of Medicine.* The chapter also documents the outcome of the vote in Virginia in 2000, when nurses won the vote for expanded prescriptive authority in the Commonwealth.

The chapter ends with one sentence summarizing the major point of the book: advanced practice nurses are professionals who can be trusted to manage their own practice at both the individual and organizational levels. That trust developed between individual doctors and nurses working at the grassroots level throughout the course of the twentieth century. It is time that this same level of trust is developed at the organizational level and that the realities of advanced practice nursing be reflected in state laws. Hopefully, this book is a step in that direction.

## Research Methods and Sources

A social history framework was used to conduct this research. Primary sources included the Lillian Wald collections at the New York Public Library and Columbia University; the Frontier Nursing Service (FNS) collection at the University of Kentucky; the FNS photographic collection at the Ekstrom Library, the University of Louisville; the Works Progress Administration (WPA) papers at the Kornhauser Library at the University of Louisville; the Virginia Brown, Ida Bahl, and Lillian Watson collection at Northern Arizona University; the Bureau of Indian Affairs papers housed at the National Archives and Records Administration in Washington, DC.; the American Association of Nurse Anesthetists papers in Chicago; and medical and nursing journals of the particular decades. In addition, the following collections were also consulted: the Bethany Hospital Coronary Care Unit (CCU) collection, Kansas City; the Joan E. Lynaugh photographic collection, The Center for the Study of the History of Nursing, and the Main Presbyterian Hospital collection, University of Pennsylvania; the National Association of Pediatric Nurse Associates and Practitioners (NAPNAP) papers, the National Certification Board of Pediatric Nurse Practitioner's collection, the Rose Pinneo collection, the Joanne Peach collection, the Barbara Brodie Collection, and the Arlene Keeling collection, all at the Center for Nursing Historical Inquiry (CNHI), the University of Virginia. Oral histories with several nurse practitioners were also done, the transcripts of which are located in the Keeling Collection, CNHI.

CHAPTER 1

# Midway between the Pharmacist and the Physician

## The Work of the Henry Street Settlement Visiting Nurses, 1893–1944

1929

Ellis M. Black, MD
Chair of the Medical Economic Committee,
Westchester Medical Group, New York

My dear Dr. Black:

Your letter as Chairman of the Westchester Village Medical Group
addressed to Miss Elizabeth Neary, Supervisor of our Westchester
Office, has been referred to me for reply. May I call the attention of
your group to the fact that in administering the work in that office,
Miss Neary does so as a representative of the Henry Street
Settlement Visiting Nurse Service and in accord with definite policies in effect throughout the entire city-wide service. It has been the
unvarying policy of the organization over the 35 years of its service
to work in close cooperation with the medical profession doing
nursing and preventive health work entirely and avoiding any sem-
blance of the "practice of medicine in competition with the doctors." . . .
[We] will call a meeting . . . to which the members of your group
will be invited for a frank discussion of our common problems.

Very truly yours,
Elizabeth Mackenzie,
Associate Director of Nurses[1]
[Henry Street Settlement, New York]

1

In 1929, Elizabeth J. Mackenzie, associate director of nurses for the Henry Street Settlement (HSS), wrote this letter to the chair of the Medical Economic Committee of the Westchester Village Medical Group, clearly stating her disapproval of the medical group's accusation that the Henry Street Visiting Nurses were practicing medicine—that is, diagnosing conditions and prescribing medicines. The Henry Street Settlement had been in existence since 1893, and its visiting nurses had been providing care on the Lower East Side of New York City for over thirty-five years. During that time the nurses had attended to a plethora of ills, including poverty, overcrowded and filthy living conditions, child labor, sweat shops, contaminated milk and water supplies, infectious disease, and high infant mortality.[2] Since 1919, Henry Street nurses had also been working uptown in the Bronx, caring not only for the poor, but also for middle-class families who had fallen on hard times. During the 1920s, the Bronx medical society had occasionally questioned whether the nurses' work was outside nursing's scope of practice (as defined by the New York state nurse practice act); but by 1928, after several meetings with the Henry Street nurses, the medical society had been referring more indigent patients to them. Now, in 1929, with the collapse of the American economy, the Westchester Village Medical Group, a constituent of the Bronx medical society, was again protesting their work. The doctors particularly opposed the well-baby conferences that the nurses conducted. Their grounds were that the nurses were practicing medicine and "entering into economic competition with them."[3]

Clearly irritated by the accusations, Elizabeth Mackenzie argued in her letter that the well-baby conferences (clinics) were solely for the purpose of health instruction for mothers with infants and preschool children, although she conceded that the nurses gave complete physical exams and immunizations. Defending the nurses' work, Mackenzie pointed out that a "careful study of the financial standing of the patients attending these conferences" shows them unable to meet the regular charges by physicians for these types of services."[4] In other words, if the HSS nurses had *not* provided care in these clinics, the indigent children would have gone without well-baby checkups and immunizations.

## Attending Patients in the Home

In order to understand the nurses' role with regard to medications, it is important to understand the context in which these nurses worked. In addition to conducting the well-baby clinics, the HSS visiting nurses provided care for patients in their crowded tenement homes.[5] In fact, much of what the HSS nurses did was the administration of routine care commonly used by white, middle-class Americans when someone was ill. This care included bathing the patient, feeding him broths and other simple foods, changing the bed linens, and keeping the room well ventilated and clean. According to director Lillian Wald's records on the care of a patient with tuberculosis:

> February 21: Mrs. K___ confined, attended by HSS nurses. Medicine, clothing, and bed-clothing given by HSS. Also eggs and milk. . . . [6]

In this case, medications were used in conjunction with other treatments considered equally important.

The other part of the nurses' work was actually the provision of nursing care routinely given in hospitals in the early twentieth century. The administration of mustard baths and other treatments like mustard plasters, turpentine stupes, and enemas composed some of their efforts at symptomatic relief. For example, the nurses frequently gave baths [ordered by physicians as a treatment] to reduce fevers. Writing in 1902, HSS nurse Jane Hitchcock described the treatment:

> A favorite method of reducing temperature with children is the mustard tub-bath. A child's tub is filled three-fourths full with tepid water. Mustard in the proportion of one heaping tablespoonful to a gallon is added. The patient is given stimulant before being placed in the tub; ice is kept on the head and constant gentle friction is applied during immersion. The effect of these baths is felt for several hours, and hence this method has been found most satisfactory in cases where the attendants cannot be depended upon to give regularly the hourly cooling sponge bath.[7]

In addition to administering such treatments (prescribed or not), the HSS nurses also taught patients about various "positive health" steps they could take, like cleaning the house or boiling dishes contaminated with tuberculosis germs. However, more often than not these treatments remained invisible in the HSS records, as the nurses frequently summarized all of their activities in one word, noting that the patient was "attended." To the nurses, such care was routine and hardly worth mentioning.

Although the Henry Street nurses' care may have been routine, the conditions in which they practiced were not. Rats, mice, and roaches complicated the HSS nurses' work. The vermin also deterred the nurses from taking the night shift. According to one nurse:

Peter had pneumonia, complicated with whooping cough. He is a beautiful yellow-haired boy, and even if the hospital could have admitted him, or his mother would have agreed to his removal (which she wouldn't), I should not have liked to send him. . . . The doctor had ordered bath treatments every two hours. These I gave until eight o'clock and the mother continued them . . . but when the tempera-ture was highest she was worn out and active night-nursing seemed imperative .·. . a service more difficult than it appears in the mere telling, for the vermin in these houses are horribly active at night.[8]

## Cultural Sensitivity

In all cases, the HSS nurses were challenged to understand cultural differ-ences. In New York City in the early years of the twentieth century, the nurses—white and middle- to upper-class—came face to face with the health beliefs and cultures of the Irish, Italian, Polish, Russian, Hungarian, African Americans, and others. Typical of the HSS nurses, who were often shocked by what they saw, Lavinia Dock wrote:

. . . the fear of bathing and of air, so deeply grounded in European medical teaching, as it would appear, is universal among our foreign people, and it is a most piteous sight to come into a small, stuffy, crowded room, with every window tightly closed, and find a child blazing with scarlet [fever] or measles, with inflamed eyes, occluded nostrils, and angry throat, pasty and sticky with the dirt of a week upon him, and dressed in full woolen clothing, shoes and stockings, and an enormous scarf or towel swathed around his poor little neck, with probably a slice of greasy bacon tied underneath. The bed is invariably filthy, for the parents are afraid to annoy him.[9]

Despite their shock, the nurses attempted to be as sensitive to the cul-tural and health beliefs of the immigrant families as their upbringing would allow. Moreover, the nurses were often assigned to work with the specific group with whom they could best relate. For example, according to 1901 HSS head nurse Jane Hitchcock: "Each nurses' personal taste is considered and the one who finds herself most in sympathy with the Irish people is sent to an Irish district, the Jewish to a Jewish, the Bohemian to a Bohemian, etc."[10] While not willing to forgo teaching the immigrants American middle-class values, the HSS nurses were nonetheless willing to meet them halfway in order to establish a sense of trust. Hitchcock reserved judgment when she reported on one case:

The world in general has a mistaken idea that poverty is synonymous with dirt and squalor. While order and cleanliness, according to our standards, are hard to attain by the woman who must be wife, mother, cook, nurse-maid, and laundress all in one, they are often found to a remarkable degree. . . . This little kitchen into which the nurse entered shows thrift and cleanliness in its furnishings. There is disorder, true, but illness, a large family and the early hour give explanation. . . . The third door leads into the bedroom proper . . . the smallest of the three [rooms], with its one window opening into the airshaft. The bed fills just three-quarters of the room space . . . pushed into the corner, it is impossible to pass around it, and all work has to be done from the one exposed side. . . . With tactful suggestions from the nurse, the mother begins to see what help she can give. . . . After a couple of days a fairly orderly routine is established, windows are coaxed open, the mother or friends have learned many little procedures and often develop a surprising quickness at learning.[11]

Nonetheless, Hitchcock's biases show through as she notes that she is surprised (probably because of their language barriers and poverty) by their level of intelligence.

## The Origins of the Henry Street Settlement

Nurses' *de facto* prescriptive care for the underprivileged on the Lower East Side began in 1893, when the settlement was first organized. In the last decades of the nineteenth century and well into the 1920s, immigration from Europe was at its peak. Thousands of Polish, Irish, Italian, Jewish, and Russian immigrants moved into the densely populated cities of the northeastern United States, trying to start a new life in America. Life in the congested cities was difficult for the poor. Racism, the rise of big business, and the distribution of wealth into the hands of a few spawned numerous social problems. Housing was expensive, and many immigrants crowded into tenements, typically with whole families and their rent-paying boarders sharing one tiny flat. Outside, the streets were littered with filth.

There was no plan for garbage collection, nor were there adequate drainage or sewage systems. As a result, the roads were a quagmire of mud and water, and uncollected garbage lined their edges. Conditions in the workplace were no better. Lower-class immigrant parents and their children, some as young as six or eight years old, worked long hours in poorly lit and unventilated factories and sweat shops. Many poor women did piecework in their homes in an attempt to make extra income. Sometimes the women themselves were sick with tuberculosis when they handled the garments they were piecing; other times, the women piled fabrics on beds or tables in the same room as their infected children.[12] Under these conditions, epidemics of infectious diseases were commonplace.

In 1893 Lillian Wald, a well-to-do, young graduate nurse from the elite New York Training School for Nurses, and her colleague Mary Brewster established the Henry Street Settlement House with the financial backing of philanthropist Jacob H. Schiff. Before that time, Wald had spent two years in a New York Training School for Nurses and supplemented that education with classes at a medical college. Wald described its origins in an article later published in the *American Journal of Nursing*:

> About eight years ago tenement-house life in its most pitiable aspect was presented to me. I had been giving a course of lessons in home nursing to a group of proletariats from the older world—people who find a renewal of hope in New York. . . . One morning one of the women of the class was not present, and her little daughter came to ask me to call upon her mother, as she was ill. Despite my experience in a large metropolitan hospital, and the subsequent knowledge gained through a year's residence in a reformatory . . . , the exposure of that rear tenement in the lower East Side was a most terrible shock. . . . A picture was presented of human creatures, moral, and in so far as their opportunities allowed them, decent members of society, . . . up dirty steps into a sick-room where there was no window, the one opening leading into a small crowded room where husband, children and boarders were gathered together . . . impossible conditions . . . to me personally it was a call to live near such conditions; to use what power an individual may possess as a citizen to help them. . . . To a friend [Mary Brewster] the plan was revealed: "Let us two nurses move into that neighborhood; let us give our services as nurses." Having formulated some necessary details of the plan, we proceeded to look for suitable quarters and in the search discovered the "settlement." For the first two months of our experiment we two nurses lived at the College Settlement. After that the top floor of a tenement that gave reasonable comfort was our home for two years.[13] . . . After that, Mr. Jacob H. Schiff [a wealthy banker and philanthropist], who from the very beginning had made us feel his support, encouragement, and confidence, suggested the change from the tenement quarters to a house, arguing that a more permanent basis would be established for these personal services if it were made possible for others to join us."[14]

After two years working from the tenement flat, Lillian Wald and Mary Brewster moved to a house at 265 Henry Street and set up headquarters for the settlement there. From its inception in 1893 until 1944, when the social and nursing activities were separated, the Henry Street Settlement (HSS) linked nursing, social welfare, and the public.[15] In addition to providing social services such as kindergartens, study rooms, playgrounds, Boys' and Girls' Clubs, and summer camps, the Henry Street Settlement was unique in its operation of a visiting nurse service that provided skilled, professional nursing care to the thousands of immigrants who crowded into the ethnic ghettos of the city.[16]

During the decades following 1900, the HSS nurses' practice expanded as they cared for patients with a multitude of illnesses. According to Wald, the needs of these New York City residents were limitless:

> There were nursing infants, many of them with the summer bowel complaint that sent infant mortality soaring during the hot months; there were children with measles, not quarantined; there were children with opthalmia, a contagious eye disease; there were children scarred with vermin bites; there were adults with typhoid; there was a case of puerperal septicemia, lying on a vermin-infested bed without sheets or pillow cases; a family consisting of a pregnant mother, a crippled child and two others living on dry bread . . . ; a young girl dying of tuberculosis amid the very conditions that had produced the disease.[17]

Initially Lillian Wald and Mary Brewster responded to these needs themselves, operating from their small flat on the Lower East Side and visiting families in their immediate neighborhood. They bathed patients, gave medicines (both home remedies and those ordered by physicians) and food, changed bed linens, and taught families to burn trash and sweep their apartments. Convinced that "the sickness they encountered in families was part of a larger set of social problems, Wald immediately began to mobilize an impressive . . . array of services . . . to provide patients with ice, sterilized milk, medicines [from their central medicine chest], meals, and referrals to many of the city's hospitals, dispensaries, and, most important, jobs."[18] By 1895 Wald and Brewster had expanded their staff to include a powerful group of nurses, including Lavinia Dock, Adelaide Nutting, and Annie Goodrich, all of whom would go on to be leaders in the profession.

By 1900 the settlement employed twelve nurses "regularly engaged in systematic visiting nursing" and made 26,600 calls.[19] Most of these calls were for acute cases, including pneumonia, typhoid, scarlet fever, and diphtheria—and nurses gave the care, administering both home remedies and prescription drugs.[20]

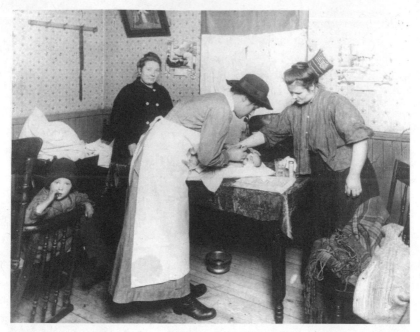

Figure 1.1: A visiting nurse on call, date unknown. Courtesy of The Visiting Nurse Service of New York

By 1909, the nursing service was outgrowing 265 Henry Street. The service now had eleven houses throughout the city and the HSS nurses began to live in flats of their own in the neighborhoods where they worked, rather than in the main headquarters on Henry Street.[21] Some lived in Harlem, the northwest section of the city that housed the majority of the African American community. Just eight years earlier, in 1901, the settlement had expanded its work to include African Americans. That year the HSS had hired Jessie Sleet, an African American nurse who had been trained at Providence Hospital in Chicago, to work in an experimental role caring for patients in the "Negro" district. The HSS later expanded its visiting nurse services to include the Stillman House Branch of the Henry Street Settlement for Colored People in a small store on West Sixty-First Street, part of the San Juan Hill area on the west side of Manhattan. Working within the confines of a racist society, four black nurses visited sick black patients, who, after years of racism, poverty, and oppression, often distrusted white health care professionals.[22] In 1918 these nurses made 33,024 home visits, routinely administering medicines as part of their care.[23]

## Caring for the Middle Class

By 1909, the Henry Street visiting nurses also expanded their work to include middle-class patients. That year Lillian Wald approached the Metropolitan Life Insurance Company with a proposal that involved HSS nurses. Until this time, charitable donations from affluent friends, revenues from fund-raising events, endowments, and "the occasional paying patient," had kept the Henry Street VNS in business.[24] However, as increasing numbers of families requested help, Wald turned to the Metropolitan Life Insurance Company with her proposal: she and her nurses would visit working- and middle-class patients for a small fee of fifty cents per visit. According to Wald, if Metropolitan Life would pay this modest fee, the company could "reduce the number of death benefits it paid."[25] In the spring of 1909, "a firm handshake sealed a contract between Haley Fiske, vice-president of the Metropolitan Life Insurance Company (MLI) and Lillian Wald. . . . The contract stated that, for a period of three months, trained nurses from HSS would provide health teaching and home care to MLI policyholders within a section of New York City. In return, Metropolitan agreed to pay the nurses fifty cents for each visit."[26]

Implementing this payment system was another problem. Patients themselves could request to have a *nurse* come, but if a nurse rather than a doctor visited the patients, something had to be done to cover their work legally, since nurses were not allowed to diagnose and prescribe.[27] The solution was relatively simple. Physicians wrote "standing orders" that guided the nurses' work. Backed by these orders, the nurses could treat patients. They could also refer patients to physicians and vice versa.

Within four years, HSS nurses were seeing thousands of patients each month. Their care involved both patient assessment and treatment, including medications that the nurses carried with them in their black bags. Over the next decade, the service grew exponentially. In 1923 alone, the visiting nurses made 37,262 visits and ministered to 52,126 patients.[28] They cared for patients with a wide variety of acute illnesses, including "pneumonia, typhoid fever, dysentery, thrush, colitis, scarlet fever, whooping cough, polio, influenza, diphtheria, measles, mumps, bronchitis, enteritis, tonsillitis, nephritis, burns, rheumatism, alcoholism, meningitis, tuberculosis, cardiac problems, and those with ulcers and eye diseases. In addition, the HSS nurses visited obstetrical cases, following both mother and baby over several weeks postpartum."[29] By 1924 the VNS employed 253 nurses, each averaging eight visits a day, and charging a fee of "$1.15 per visit for those who could afford it and a sliding scale or free service" for those who could not.[30] By 1926 the VNS was making over

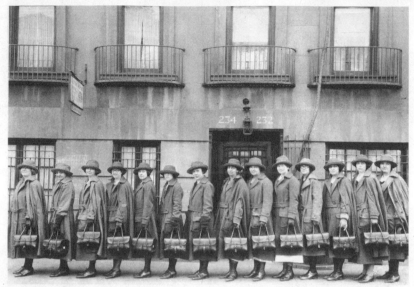

Figure 1.2: Nurses in a row, date unknown. Courtesy of The Visiting Nurse Service of New York

300,000 visits each year.[31] Thus, for years the HSS visiting nurses had been trusted and their work welcomed. Now, in 1929, when the Westchester physicians saw the nurses' work as a threat to their incomes, it was not.

## Medicine in the Progressive Era

The situation between the medical group and the HSS nurses was more complicated than a simple economic issue, however. The twentieth century was a transitional period in American medicine. Throughout the country, university-educated physicians were trying to gain control of the practice of medicine and the educational requirements for practice. The trend had started in the late nineteenth century. Then, university-trained physicians, having accepted the germ theory of disease and Lister's work with antisepsis, began the struggle to get the public to use medicines and treatments based on scientific fact and prescribed by licensed physicians rather than using "cure-alls" prescribed by uneducated, self-proclaimed "quack" physicians. Trained physicians were particularly concerned about the false advertising of patent medicines in an unrestricted market. Some of the patent drugs were simply useless, but others contained "highly addictive substances like opium, cocaine and . . . acetanilide."[32]

So the doctors were justified in their concern about the qualifications of those who prescribed medicines. Almost any man who had the money and time to complete a short apprenticeship with a physician could claim that he, too, was a physician. The medical profession was also justified in its concern about the widespread availability and misuse of the addictive drugs and their serious negative side effects. In some parts of the country, where there were few physicians, almost anyone could sell "cure-all" medicines in unlabeled bottles. The public was also concerned because there were reports of lower-class mothers drugging their infants in order to get them to sleep while the mothers worked.[33] In order to protect the public, the medical establishment demanded that the contents of patent medicines be identified and listed on the label. The profession's efforts culminated in legislative action. On June 30, 1906, President Theodore Roosevelt signed the Food and Drug Act into law, requiring true statements on medication labels and the disclosure of "alcohol, opium, cocaine, morphine, chloroform, marijuana, acetanilide, chloral hydrate or eucaine" as contents.[34] However, the 1906 Food and Drug Act did not restrict pharmacists from dispensing these over-the-counter remedies, nor did it restrict the public (at least the classes who could afford to) from purchasing them and keeping them at home.

During this time period, the few drugs available to treat illnesses were widely accessible through corner drugstores, dispensed by pharmacists to those who could afford them. There was little difference between commonly available household remedies and medical prescriptions, both of which provided symptomatic relief.[35] Medical therapies and nursing care were often identical, as well. Drugs such as cough medicines, analgesics (for pain), and antipyretics (for fever), used in conjunction with skilled nursing care, frequently composed standard medical treatment.

## Working in the Middle

The HSS nurses used both physician-prescribed medications and middle-class household remedies as they attended lower-class patients and their families. In essence, they practiced somewhere in the middle, between pharmacists and physicians, between domestic care and professional care. For centuries, but particularly since the founding of the American Medical Association (AMA) in 1847, physicians had claimed the right to prescribe medicines as solely within their professional boundaries. Pharmacists were to prepare and dispense drugs, but not to counsel patients about them. After the establishment of professional nursing in 1872, student nurses and their hospital supervisors administered physician-prescribed drugs and therapies.[36]

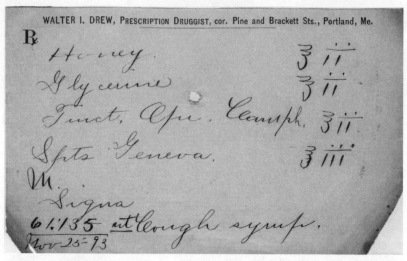

Figure 1.3: Original prescription, 1893: "honey, glycerine and sodium bicarbonate." KC, CNHI

At night and on weekends, however, if there were no pharmacist available in the hospital, nursing supervisors would also dispense medications, pouring them from larger bottles to smaller ones or from a large bottle to an individual medicine cup. The boundaries of nursing fluctuated with changing needs: nurses' scope of practice increased when the sun went down and on weekends, when other professionals were unavailable. Their scope of practice also expanded when they practiced outside the hospital among the poor.

So, from the 1840s through the 1930s, the roles of pharmacist, physician, and nurse were, as physician Albert T. Lytle put it in his 1905 address to the New York State Nurses Association, "hopelessly entangled."[37] The roles of these professionals became even more muddled when the HSS began to employ graduate nurses to provide skilled care in patients' homes. According to Lytle, nurses occupied "in reference to materia medica, pharmacy and therapeutics, and the patient, a field midway between the pharmacist and the physicians."[38]

The public's self-administration of drugs further complicated the situation, as many middle- and upper-class women kept on hand many of the same drugs that might be prescribed by physicians. Thus, practicing between domestic care and professional medical care, the nurses worked in "the middle place."[39] According to a 1903 *American Journal of Nursing* article, a home medicine closet would typically contain "Listerine, alcohol, glycerine, Pond's extract, brandy, lime-water . . . boracic acid powder, flaxseed meal, whiskey, spirits of ammonia, camphor, castor oil, turpen-

tine, chloroform liniment, arnica, camphorated oil, mustard leaves . . .
ichthyol . . . bicarbonate of soda . . . tablets of quinine, Frazer's migraine
for headache . . . cascara, soda mint, calomel, essence of peppermint,
Jamaica ginger, syrup of ipecac, paregoric . . . lavender salts, iodine, laudanum, carbolic acid, oil of clove and calomel,"[40] the same remedies prescribed by physicians, dispensed by pharmacists, carried by the nurses in
their bags, and discussed in medical and nursing textbooks.

## Prescriptions for Care

Some of the patients and families visited by the HSS nurses could not self-
medicate. They either didn't have the money to buy drugs, or they didn't
have the knowledge and skill to take care of themselves when they were ill.
In those cases, the physician's prescription might be to provide a nurse. In
fact, in the Henry Street Settlement district, physicians' requests for nursing care usually came hastily written on a prescription blank brought by a
sympathizing neighbor.

> **Rx:** Dear Miss Wald: Kindly send one of your nurses to attend baby
> ___,
> 204 ___Street, top, front, right; pneumonia. The family is poor and
> unable to give proper care.[41]

The implication was, of course, that had it been of middle- or upper-class
means, the family would have been able to afford the necessary remedies
and would have had the knowledge and skills to do so, or as Wald put it,
" . . . if the mothers had sufficient leisure or sufficient intelligence."[42] For
those who did not, the HSS visiting nurses would provide access to that
"proper care." Physicians trusted the nurses to do so. The nurses were
equipped not only with the necessary medicines, but also with the professional training needed to administer them. One nurse described that
"proper care":

> In amongst these pillows, covered by some and completely surround-
> ed by others, is the patient, a child of two years. The temperature is
> 104.5 degrees, pulse 140, respirations 50. The fair curly hair is tan-
> gled and matted, the face and hands sticky with syrupy medicine,
> while the feet and legs are still soiled with the dirt of the street. . . .
> The nurse now begins her work. . . . First, the pillows and feather-
> bed are removed; then the baby's over-abundant clothing is laid aside.
> . . . Next the cleansing soap and water bath is given, one of the cots

in the front room put into correct position as to light and air . . . and the little one laid there clean and refreshed. . . . All this is preliminary to the more definite nursing work, which includes showing the mother how to give the alcohol sponge-bath, swab the mouth, arrange the ice-caps for the head, warm bottles if necessary for the feet, and give the medicines and nourishment. Simple bedside notes are left for the doctor, showing the temperature, pulse and respiration, the general condition of the child, with a record of the work done by the nurse.[43]

Clearly, nursing care—bathing and feeding the baby, sponging him with alcohol, recording observations—was just as important as the drugs available at this time. In this case, the prescribed medicine was most likely a "pulmonary sedative" such as "codeine, hydrated chloral, bromides . . . belladonna or wild cherry," discussed in the 1903 *Physicians' Handy Book of Materia Medica,* and described by HSS nurse leader Lavinia Lloyd Dock in the 1921 edition of her *Materia Medica for Nurses.*[44]

In many instances, drugs were applied externally. For example, care of a baby with measles included "general care, mustard baths, saline enemata, camphorated oil applied to chest."[45] Prior to the advent of pills containing ephedrine [to relieve nasal congestion] and diphenhydramine [an antihistamine used to treat colds], physicians and nurses gave mustard baths and applied camphorated oil and plasters to relieve pulmonary congestion. Registered Nurse Nora Nagle discussed the use of mustard as a therapy, writing:

> Mustard, as a counter irritant, has long been used both by the medical profession and the laity. Easily obtained and easily applied, it has been used with good effect in the hospital and the home . . . in such conditions as a beginning bronchitis, (1) to relieve the congestion . . . and (2) to ward off an attack of asthma.[46]

## Bridging the Gap in Access to Medical Care

Bridging the gap between rich and poor, the HSS visiting nurses applied such measures even in cases where there was no physician available to order the treatment.[47]

Lillian Wald, who founded public health nursing while directing the Henry Street Settlement, believed that access to nursing care should not depend on patients being connected with certain physicians or hospitals. According to Wald, nurses should respond to calls from individual

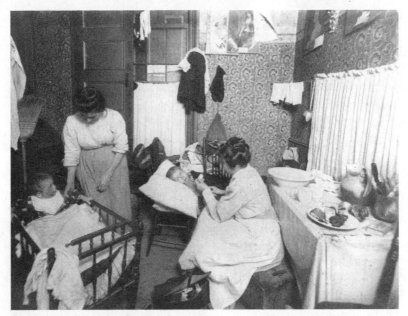

Figure 1.4: Visiting nurse with family in tenement. Visiting Nurse Society of Philadelphia Records. CSHN. The University of Pennsylvania

patients and physicians unencumbered by red tape or formality.[48] In fact, she went on to say that "a child capable of giving the address or with a slip of paper in his hand giving the address of a sick person, will procure the nurse."[49] A 1906 report on the HSS nurses' work confirmed that Wald's belief was policy at Henry Street. More than half the 5,334 patients the HSS nurses visited that year were referred by families and only 1,648 by physicians.[50] Discussing the polio epidemic in a speech to the American Academy of Medicine in 1917, Wald again reflected on the referral process, noting, "Very sick children were referred to the Settlement for care by many sources; last summer, drivers would get down from their trucks to tell of a case of poliomyelitis."[51]

Because of this referral system, it was not uncommon for an HSS nurse to observe signs and symptoms, make a presumptive (though unwritten) diagnosis, and begin treatment on her own before referring the case to a physician. According to historian Karen Buhler-Wilkerson, a "nursing visit usually preceded a call to the doctor, with the nurse deciding if the patient needed medical assistance at a dispensary, 'uptown specialist,' or hospital care."[52]

Sometimes the HSS nurses responded to the immigrants' needs by teaching them the skills middle- and upper-class mothers learned from

their own mothers or from popular magazines like *Godey's Lady's Book*.[53]
For example, in a 1916 advertisement for a course in home health nursing, the HSS nurses noted that on "Wednesday evening, December 14th at
8:00 PM," the nurses would discuss "uses of moist and dry heat, and how
to make and apply flaxseed poultices, fomentations, hot salt bags, hop
bags, turpentine stupes etc." They also advertised that "on Wednesday,
January 4, at 8:00 PM" they would teach "How to apply iodine, lini-
ments, plasters and lotions."[54] Nurses, physicians, and the lay public all
used these remedies as therapeutic treatments to provide symptomatic
relief. Besides being available in the ladies' magazines, information about
these therapies was included in both nursing textbooks of the era and the
AMA publication on medical prescriptions.[55]

## The Nurse's Bag and the Central Medicine Chest

To carry supplies to the tenement homes in their district, the HSS visiting nurses used their black bags, the "District Bags" lent to the HSS
nurses for a deposit of two dollars. These were "fully equipped except
for bandage scissors, small scissors, probe, forceps and hypodermic:
which the nurses were requested to provide."[56] Besides such articles as
these and bowls, towels, dressings, and thermometers, the bag also
included:

> One three-ounce bottle for alcohol; five one-ounce bottles contain-
> ing respectively—Listerine, whiskey, glycerine, tincture of green
> soap, and carbolic acid, 95%; one wide-mouthed bottle with
> screw-top for bichloride tablets; one one-ounce wide-mouthed bot-
> tle with screw-top for boracic acid powder; small screw-top bottle
> for cascara tablets; one two-ounce porcelain jar containing boric
> acid unguent; two one-ounce porcelain jars with ichthyol unguent,
> 10%; and Thiersch powder; one . . . jar for special dressing con-
> taining iodoform, balsam Peru etc; half ounce porcelain jar for
> Vaseline. . . . [57]

The district bag also contained "a small box of cocoa . . . a jar of beef
extract, fresh eggs for eggnog and albumin lemonade . . . and 'jellies for
the convalescents.'"[58]

Most of these medicines were household remedies, like counterirritants
and antiseptics. Listerine, for example, was a mouthwash antiseptic.
Icthyol was an ointment commonly used "to aid in the healing of
wounds," and iodoform, a gauze containing iodine, was used to pack can-

cer wounds. Thiersch powder was a "combination of salicylic and boric acids, usually added to one quart of water to form an antiseptic solution."[59] Balsam of Peru was a "vascular stimulant and nerve sedative, antiseptic and disinfectant, used externally as an application to stimulate granulating surfaces [wound healing]."[60] Both bichloride tablets and boric acid were antiseptic solutions, used to stem the growth of microbes. Other solutions were disinfectants, like carbolic acid. Green soap was a strong lye soap used to bathe patients, particularly those with lice or scabies. Some household remedies contained alcohol—whiskey was commonly used as a stimulant and analgesic. Others were narcotics—paregoric, for example, was "camphorated tincture of opium," a drug that was often used to relieve colic in infants and was, in fact, one of the problem drugs that physicians wanted to regulate. Still other drugs, like turpentine, chloroform, and mustard, were classified as "counterirritants," or "rubefacients," which turned the skin red. Caustics included silver nitrate, to be used as an eye medication. Ammonia and kerosene oil were considered vesicants and were used externally.[61] All of these home remedies were widely available—including the narcotics.

In addition to these standard ointments, solutions, and powders (many of which could be found in the medicine cabinets of middle- and upper-class families), the HSS nurses could select other medications they needed. The bags contained: "1 large bottle, 4 small bottles, 1 blue bottle and 2 tall screw-top jars"—to be filled from the HSS medicine chest at the nurses' discretion," and "1 medicine dropper and 1 syringe."[62] Filling these bottles themselves prior to making rounds each day, the nurses were assured that they had what they needed.

The HSS nurses did not always work alone, but they always used the medicine closet for their supplies. When a nurses worked in collaboration with a physician instead of on her own, she would meet the doctor

> in the early morning . . . at the stated hour to report on the cases visited the previous afternoon and that morning; receive orders and instructions for them or the new cases that he desires her to see; replenish her bag from the loan chest and medicine chest and recommence her rounds.[63]

Although the contents of the central medicine chest are not identified specifically in the HSS records, it is very likely that it contained many of the drugs listed in Dock's *Materia Medica,* which was in its seventh edition in 1921. These may have included nitroglycerine for heart patients, aspirin, castor oil, cascara (laxative), sulphur, magnesium oxide (milk of magnesia), and belladonna (atropine), a heart stimulant.[64] By the 1930s,

| Drug Supplies | Used during 1931 | Am't now on hand at Tapawingo | Order for 1932 | Check Here |
|---|---|---|---|---|
| Witch Hazel | 2 qts. | — | 2 qts. | |
| Alcohol - (70% for sponging) | 3 pints | — | 3 pints | |
| Hydrogen Peroxide | 4-ozs. | 4. ozs. | — | |
| Green Soap (full strength) | 3/4 pint | 1/4 pint | 1 Pint | |
| Agarol | 6-ozs. | — | 6-ozs. | |
| Milk of Magnesia | 3-(12 oz bottles) | — | 3 - (12 oz bottles) | |
| Castor-oil | 0 | 6- ozs. | | |
| Epsom Salts (wet dressings) | 1 lb. | — | 1-lb. | |
| Arom. Fld. Ext. of Cascara | 9-ozs. | 3-ozs | 10- ozs. | |
| Phenolax Tabs. | 5½ bottles (50 each) | ½ bottle | 6 bottles - (50 each) | |
| Lysol - (Pure) | 1½ pints | ½ Pint | 2 Pints | |
| Larkspur | 3/4 large bottle | 1/4 bottle | 1 large Bottle | |
| Tr. Iodine | 8-ozs. (ran short) | — | 10- ozs. | |
| Mercurochrome | 12-ozs. | 2 ozs. | 14- ozs. | |
| Argyrol - 10% | 3-ozs. | — | 4. ozs. | |
| Rhubarb & Soda Mixture | 13-ozs. | 1-oz. | 14. ozs. | |
| Brown Mixture | 16-ozs. | — | 12. ozs. | |
| Elixir Terpin Hydrate | 4-ozs. | — | 6-ozs. | |
| Zinc Oxide Ointment | 1 Tube | — | 1 Tube | |
| Zonite " | 8 " | — | 6 " | |
| Icthyol " | 2 " | — | 2 " | |
| Vaseline (White) | 1/4 Jar | 3/4 Jar | — | |
| Unguentine | 4 Tubes | ½ Tube | 4 Tubes | |
| Vicks - Vapo-rub | 1½ Jar | ½ Jar | 2 Jars. | |

Figure 1.5: Drugs and Supplies: Camp Tapawingo, 1931. Lillian Wald Collection, Rare Book and Manuscript Library, Butler Library, Columbia University

the medicine chest probably contained many of the drugs kept in stock at Camp Tapawingo, one of the summer camps operated by the Henry Street Settlement.[65] Among numerous others, these included: tincture of iodine for the "disinfection and treatment of wounds"[66]; zinc oxide ointment (used for diaper rash); rhubarb and soda, for "strengthening appetite and digestion"[67]; cascara (a "laxative and cathartic")[68]; and elixir of terpin hydrate, a cough medicine made from oil of turpentine.

From this wide assortment of remedies, the visiting nurses could choose different drugs based on the patient needs they anticipated on any

given day. No doubt they were well supplied. Next to gauze dressings, car-
fare, and telephone, "drugs and supplies" were a significant expenditure of
the organization.[69]

## Necessary Knowledge for Safe Care

In the early twentieth century, nurses were legally responsible for the safe
administration of prescribed drugs,[70] and the Henry Street nurses knew a
great deal about drugs. From the inception of professional nursing education in the late nineteenth century, nurses had been learning about *materia medica* and administering medications to their patients. In the late
1880s, for example, student nurses were taught about giving "opium, amyl
nitrate, tincture of iodine, and calomel, as well as Turpentine stupes."[71] In
addition, they were taught the uses and administration of laudanum and
digitalis, as well as the proper technique for administering injections.
Nurses were also instructed that "whiskey, brandy, liquid ammonia, nitrate
of amyl, atropia, belladonna, caffeine, cocaine, mustard, sulphide of zinc,
Gallic acid, ergot and pilocarpine," should be kept "on hand."[72] By the
time the Henry Street Settlement opened in the 1890s and these drugs
were used, the nurses were familiar with them.

In addition, the Henry Street Settlement nurses were required to have
post-RN training in public health nursing before they could work as visiting
nurses. They had already had introductory *materia medica* in their training
programs and now had further education about pharmacy in the public
health curriculum. They were also taught how to care for patients in their
homes and what to teach them so that the patients might take care of themselves. Even after they took the prerequisite public health nurses training, the
nurses took advantage of continuing educational opportunities. As Lillian
Wald noted in a 1921 speech at Columbia University, many of the nurses
already held degrees from leading colleges and universities . . . but were
"availing themselves of the courses open to them because of [the settlement's]
affiliation with Columbia University."[73] Clearly, these were not average hospital staff nurses. They were experienced, well-educated nurses who had sufficient and necessary knowledge to provide safe care.

## De Facto Diagnosing

The HSS visiting nurse was often the first professional to see a patient.
Consequently, she was the one who made an initial, though tentative, diagnosis. In fact, HSS nurses routinely diagnosed common health problems

like ear infections, diarrhea, and thrush as they made "sick rounds" throughout the tenement districts.[74] In one case, an HSS nurse diagnosed and treated a child and then referred him to a physician for follow-up. Visiting a second child, she administered a commonly used home remedy for diarrhea. Then, visiting a third household, the nurse gave the mother another household treatment for her baby's sore mouth.

> In one room, I found a child with running ears which I syringed, showing the mother how to do it, and directed her to Dr. Koplik of Essex Street Dispensary for further treatment. . . . In another room, a child with summer complaint to whom I gave bismuth and tickets for a sea-side excursion. . . . On the next floor, the Castria baby had a sore mouth for which I gave the mother borax and honey and little cloths to keep it clean.[75]

During their home visits, HSS nurses observed and interpreted various signs and symptoms and took the required action, despite the fact that by law they were not allowed to diagnose. A 1934 *American Journal of Public Health* article described their reality:

> It is not the essential purpose of the [public health] nurse to make definite diagnoses, nor necessarily to treat patients of her own initiative. . . . Despite this principle, obviously it is impossible to avoid making some diagnoses. To recognize measles, pediculosis, caries, kyphosis, conjunctivitis and similar conditions is not only difficult to avoid, but it is immediately desirable, in order to institute promptly the necessary measures for the protection of the rest of the family and community.[76]

In the absence of the physician, HSS nurses did what they needed to do. They had no choice. If they were to provide safe and effective care, they had to make de facto diagnoses on which to base that care.[77]

## Prescribing?

Technically, the HSS nurses did not prescribe drugs for their patients. That is, they did not write prescriptions for medications to be filled at a drugstore. The 1903 statute regulating the registration of nurses in New York was explicit:

> Before beginning to practice nursing every registered nurse shall cause such certificate to be recorded in the county clerk's office of the

county of . . . her residence with an affidavit of . . . her identity as the person to whom the same was so issued. . . . Nothing contained in this act shall be considered as conferring any authority to practice medicine or to undertake the treatment or cure of disease.[78]

According to tradition and the law, "the treatment and cure of disease" included prescribing medicines, and this was to be done by physicians.[79] In a 1906 *American Journal of Nursing* article, Albert Lytle, MD, was unequivocal in his remarks to nurses about their role in relationship to medications, reinforcing the law: "the nurse only administers [drugs] and neither prescribes nor dispenses."[80] Regulation #14 of the HSS was equally clear, specifying that "a nurse must never prescribe for a patient."[81] And, technically, following these rules, the HSS nurses did not prescribe; they followed medical orders as was customary, giving medicines prescribed by physicians or dispensing medicines from their bags. According to one HSS record:

Child of two years—pneumonia—parent poor—dispensary physician making occasional calls and receiving daily reports from nurses. Nurse visited daily for 3 weeks, two visits a day during the critical period, giving baths . . . cleansing mouth . . . instructing family . . . [giving] drugs from dispensary.[82]

In this instance, the nurse was working cooperatively with the dispensary physician, reporting to him and giving the drugs he had prescribed. No doubt, the family had no money to fill the prescription, and the nurses, following Wald's instructions to "take the prescription and have it filled, and relieve the immediate pressure," purchased the drugs herself and administered them to the patient.[83]

It was not only the medical profession's ownership of the prescriptive privilege that limited nurses' legal autonomy in practice.[84] By the early twentieth century, the medical profession was increasingly assertive about its scope of practice as regulated by state laws. Both the American Medical Association and the American College of Surgeons (established in 1913) were gaining control of the profession and its practice. Furthermore, the nursing profession was not questioning their authority. In fact, quite the opposite was true. Nurse leaders were adamant that prescriptive authority was the purview of the medical profession. The preface to a set of "standing orders" for Chicago visiting nurses in 1913, which were to be "carried in the nurses' bags" and "sent to every physician carrying free cases," emphasized this regulation. According to that document, "No medication, not even castor oil, is included in this list [of standing orders] for obvious reasons."[85] Clearly, the nursing profession itself was identifying its practice boundaries, despite the practical realities.

By 1926, practice boundaries were becoming increasingly well defined. That year, in a draft of the *Code of Ethics* for the American Nurses Association, the nurse authors were unequivocal that the role of the nurse was complementary to that of the physician. The nurse was not to use her independent judgment to prescribe:

> The term "medicine" should be understood to refer to scientific medicine and the desirable relationship between the two should be one of mutual respect. The key to the situation lies in the mutuality of aim of medicine and nursing: the aims, to cure and prevent disease and promote positive health are identical, the technics [*sic*] are different and neither can secure complete results without the other. The nurse should respect the physician as the person legally and professionally responsible for the medical and surgical treatment of the patient. She should endeavor to give much intelligent and skilled nursing service that she be looked upon as a co-worker and not a handmaiden. Under no circumstances, except in an emergency, is the nurse justified in instituting therapeutic treatment.[86]

The question remained—did the care of all urban poor qualify as an emergency?

## Fluid Boundary Lines

The imaginary line separating nursing from medicine was fluid, especially when over-the-counter medicines were used. As has been noted, the HSS nurses recommended and used home remedies, which at the turn of the twentieth century were part of both professional nursing care and medical therapeutics. For example, borax glycerine (one part borax to four parts glycerine) "gently painted on four times a day" was a commonly prescribed treatment for thrush (a yeast infection commonly occurring in infants' mouths).[87] Nurses shared knowledge of this treatment with physicians. According to Shaw's 1902 *Textbook of Nursing*, treatment for thrush was "a wash of borax water."[88] Since borax and glycerine were kept in home medicine cabinets at the time, it is likely that this treatment was also widely used by the lay public; whether the HSS nurse was prescribing a medical therapy, a professional nursing treatment, or a middle- and upper-class home remedy is not clear. Nor did it seem to matter much, as long as the infant received care.

In addition to borax and glycerine, both nurses and physicians used physiologic saline, particularly as a throat irrigation in the treatment of diphtheria or scarlet fever. According to a 1926 textbook of medicine:

> When, in an infant . . . the throat becomes foul and in obvious need
> of cleansing as may occur in diphtheria or scarlet fever, there is noth-
> ing that meets the requirements as well as copious irrigation of the
> throat with hot physiologic sodium chloride solution. The infant, its
> arms confined by safety pinned blanket, is laid face down on the
> nurse's lap, and the fluid is squirted from the nozzle of a fountain
> syringe backward into the little one's throat in intervals between
> inspirations. The fluid escapes from the mouth and nose, carrying
> with it, at times, surprising quantities of mucus, pus, and necrotic
> material. The irrigation is continued until nothing further comes
> away. It is best not to add any medicament to the water as much of
> it is liable to be swallowed.[89]

Once again, the professional boundaries were fluid. In this case, the physician
prescribed a nursing treatment using physiologic saline; in practice, nurses
mixed physiologic saline according to recipes in nursing textbooks. Nurses
were familiar with this standard treatment from their training school lectures
and no doubt initiated it on their own accord when the need arose.

## Cards of Instruction in School Nursing

In addition to administering prescription drugs and initiating treatments
on their own when circumstances demanded it, the HSS nurses gave drugs
and administered therapeutic treatments according to standing orders.
Evidence of this practice is nowhere more apparent than in HSS school
nursing activities, where the nurses used "cards of instruction"—standing
orders to be implemented in the care of children with specific diagnoses.

Although physicians from the Department of Health had been inspect-
ing American schools since the mid-nineteenth century, most of their attention had focused on the identification and exclusion of children with contagious diseases. In 1903 under an experimental program in New York City,
nurses visited schools to treat children and follow up cases, with the goal of
reducing absenteeism; only "the children suffering from serious disorders
too advanced to be cared for in the dressing-room were sent home."[90]

Henry Street Settlement school nurses visited, on average, four schools
in a day, treating children who had "been selected by the doctor on his
daily rounds."[91] In her "Daily Report," HSS nurse Lina L. Rogers noted
that she treated 893 cases in October (c. 1920s) in parochial schools #147,
#12, and #31, and that these cases included "eye troubles, eczema, ring-
worm and minor wounds."[92] Each disease had its own treatment protocol
outlined by the New York City Department of Health, which was to be

"followed without variation unless the Medical Inspector prescribes some special treatment." According to those directions:

> The following methods will hereafter be used in treating children sent to the nurse by the Medical Inspector of schools:
>
> Pediculosis—Saturate head and hair with equal parts kerosene and sweet oil; next day wash with solution of potassium carbonate. . . . To remove nits, use hot vinegar.
>
> Favus (Ringworm of scalp)—Mild cases: Scrub with tincture green soap; epilate; cover with flexible collodion. Severe cases: Scrub with tincture green soap; epilate; paint with tincture iodine and cover with flexible collodion.
>
> Ringworm of face and body—Wash with tincture green soap and cover with flexible collodion.
>
> Scabies—Scrub with tincture green soap; apply sulphur ointment.
>
> Impetigo—Remove crust with tincture green soap; apply white precipitate ointment (ammonia hydrarg).
>
> Molluscum contagiosum—Express contents; apply tincture iodine on cotton toothpick probe.
>
> Conjunctivitis—Irrigate with solution of boric acid.[93]

In compliance with such standing orders, the HSS nurses provided medical treatments to the children, noting that the work was done "with the equipment of the Settlement Bag, and in some of the schools, no more than the ledge of a window and the corner of a room for the nurses' office."[94] Having treated the children, the nurse would take her list of names and "make visits in the homes after school hours," interviewing the mothers and "giving whatever advice" was needed.[95] According to school nurse Lina Rogers, the most commonly occurring conditions included contagious eye disease, pediculosis, eczema, and scabies, and school nurses had permission to treat these. They could not "at any time" treat trachoma (a serious eye infection), however, which was considered too high a "source of contagion."[96]

## Interdisciplinary Conflicts

While most physicians supported the HSS nursing activities in health promotion and the prevention of disease, not all were enamored of the visiting nurses' work, particularly in relationship to dispensing medications and treatments. In 1904 some members of the New York medical community expressed their concern that HSS nurses were in fact carrying drugs in their bags and making home visits to patients without physician referral. Word of their concern reached director Lillian Wald via a circuitous route, spreading from the downtown doctors to the uptown medical specialists and back to Wald in a letter from her friend Lavinia L. Dock, who was traveling in Europe. Writing to Wald from Paris on June 30, 1904, Dock reported the gossip she had heard about the Henry Street nurses:

> Miss Maude Banfield [a nurse colleague] has just come to visit us and she told me an incident that I must tell you at once, though you may probably have heard it all. . . . She crossed [the Atlantic] on a steamer with Mrs. Felix Adler [a New York socialite] and to my amazement, she [Adler] seems to be quite violently in opposition to you and your work in this question of the nursing [and] the doctors. When she found that Miss Banfield was a nurse she immediately entered with much energy and determination, on what she called this "question" in New York and told Miss Banfield with strong disapproval that "Miss Wald's nurses carried *ointments* in their bags and that they even *gave pills!* She is of the opinion that it is quite wrong for district nursing to be done in any way except under the strict control of the physicians—the nurses ought not to go to cases except on their orders—doctors ought to be in charge of district nursing associations—no nursing ought to be done in any other method. . . . It seems Mrs. Adler gets all these ideas from her brother-in-law who is a doctor . . . you must be on your guard against them. I don't doubt that the downtown physician's society has taken their complaints to the uptown men hoping to get there a stronger support and perhaps injure you in your finances. LLD[97]

Dock had long been aware that not all physicians were pleased with the independent aspects of the HSS visiting nurses' work, particularly the administration of medications and treatments in the First Aid Rooms that the HSS nurses established. In the first aid rooms, established within their various settlement houses, the HSS nurses treated patients for all sorts of minor conditions. They changed dressings and administered topical ointments and remedies for "innumerable burns, local infections, cuts, bumps . . . small accidents . . . eczemas of the scalp and face, conjunctivitis, and troubles common in ill-nourished children."[98] The rumors reported by Maude Banfield were true: the Henry Street nurses *did* carry ointments in their bags, *did* in fact give pills, and *did* make home visits without physician referral. They also treated thousands of patients in the first aid dispensaries.

What is interesting is that Dock does not deny these aspects of the nurses' role in her letter to Wald. She does, however, worry that the additional first aid rooms they had recently opened might also be criticized and suggests that the settlement should be sure to have standing medical orders for the care they gave, writing:

> Of course we don't practice medicine nor want to. . . . But they [the physicians] might say that our First Aid Room was a practice of medicine. . . . I think we'll have to be more careful than ever to have always some doctor's orders behind us.[99]

Clearly, the Henry Street nurses were stretching the limits of nursing practice, and Dock was concerned about the legality of their care. Having standing orders written by physicians would cover the nurses in that respect. Then the nurses could continue to provide care—that they were in fact qualified to give—to those to whom it would otherwise be denied.

## Collaboration and Cooperation

Despite the conflict noted by Dock, during the late-nineteenth and early-twentieth centuries, many of the New York physicians and the HSS nurses worked out solutions to their boundary problems. From the inception of the Settlement, numerous physicians supported the visiting nurse service. For example, physician Dr. Paul S. Kaplan, an East Side Russian doctor, cared for hundreds of Russian immigrants,[100] while imminent uptown specialists like Henry Koplik, Abraham Jacobi, Henry D. Chapman, Harry Lorner, Lollis Greenwald, and Marcus Rothschild[101] also treated the poor, accepting referrals from the Henry Street nurses.

Others supported the HSS nurses for another reason: if the nurses made home visits to the poor or saw them in the first aid rooms, the physicians could spend their time on paying patients. Early on, with the endorsement of the local medical society, the Henry Street Settlement nurses established standing orders for emergency medications and treatments to ensure the legal operation of the first aid rooms.[102] Standing orders were also implemented for school nursing. In fact, the standing orders provided a practical and convenient way for nurses to use their skills of physical assessment, planning, and implementation of care for the indigent, without bothering physicians.

In addition to working with the local medical society, the Henry Street Visiting Nurse Service established a medical advisory committee who "counseled on matters dealing with the relationship between the medical and the nursing groups and the development of policies relating to the welfare of patients."[103] That committee would be needed as a mediator between the nurses and the Westchester Village Medical group in 1929, when Elizabeth J. Mackenzie reported that "difficulties with a certain group of doctors in the Bronx," while "not new," had surfaced again.[104] The accusations were not surprising. Clearly the Westchester physicians were worried that the nurses would threaten their incomes. It was 1929, and the economic crisis that engulfed the entire nation began to focus everyone's attention on money. A few years later, in California, physician anesthesiologists also challenged the limits of nursing practice. In their case, it was nurse-anesthetists who were the focus of attention.

# CHAPTER 2

# Practicing Medicine without a License?

## Nurse Anesthetists, 1900–1938

Setting: The Superior Court of California, 1934—"Chalmers-Francis v. Nelson"

Leroy Anderson [attorney for the physicians]: You are—and I think it is admitted—you are not a registered physician or surgeon?

Dagmar Nelson, RN [the defendant]: I am not, Mr. Anderson.

Anderson: . . . Your training has been as a nurse?

Nelson: It has been.

Anderson: Yes, and you have never applied for license to practice as a physician or surgeon in California?

Nelson: I have not.

Anderson: In the giving of these anesthetics . . . you have made use of drugs in each and every one of them [the cases], have you not, Miss Nelson?

Nelson: Yes, the anesthetic generally is considered a drug.

Anderson: Will you give us the names of the drugs most usually used by you in the operations—those anesthetics that you have administered?

Nelson: Nitrous oxide, oxygen . . . carbon dioxide, ether . . .

Anderson: "All right. And you use . . . your judgment as to the amount to be administered . . . ?

Mr. Valle, [attorney for the defendant Dagmar Nelson]: Objected to on the grounds it calls for a conclusion and opinion of the witness.

Court: Sustained. . . . Reframe the question.

Anderson: . . . You use varying amounts, don't you?

Nelson: Yes.

Anderson: . . . You yourself always determine the amount to be given or not to be given, don't you?

Nelson: I do.

Anderson: . . . and you watch constantly. Then, from these observations and this constant watch that you make of the patient . . . you either give less or more of the nitrous oxide, we will say, or the carbon dioxide, or you apply the oxygen or not, is that correct?

Nelson: Yes, and also depending upon the relaxation of the patient.

Anderson: . . . under your training as a nurse, are you ever permitted to prescribe the amount of any dosage of any medicine . . . that you give?

Nelson: No.

Anderson: Does the surgeon in charge of the case while you are giving an anesthetic assist you in any way in giving that anesthetic?

Nelson: No.

Anderson: And that is in fact practicing medicine without a license, is it not?

Valee: Objection, your honor . . .[1]

Attorney Leroy Anderson was trying to prove that nurse anesthetist Dagmar A. Nelson was not qualified under the laws of California to deliver anesthesia. Arguing in the Superior Court of the State of California in 1934, Anderson, the attorney for the physicians, maintained that Nelson had not taken or passed the examination to practice medicine, nor did she have a license to practice as a physician or surgeon in California. Because she was not licensed as a physician, she could not give anesthesia: in California only physicians could prescribe drugs. Therefore, the anesthesia division of the Los Angeles County Medical Association, represented by William Chalmers-Francis, MD, was suing nurse anesthetist Dagmar Nelson and St. Vincent's Hospital for the "illegal practice of medicine in violation of the state's medical practice act."[2] This lawsuit was the third challenge to nurse anesthesia practice since 1911 and was a significant break with the general spirit of cooperation between the medical and nursing professions in the seventy-three years since the Civil War, when women volunteers and Catholic sisters assisted with anesthesia. Its outcome would set legal precedent for the practice of nurse anesthesia for the remainder of the century.

## Roots of Nurse Anesthesia

When the American Civil War began in 1861, there were few professional nurses in the country. In fact, only a few training schools had been established in the United States, some dating back to the 1830s. One of those schools, the Graduate School for Nurses in Philadelphia, had just opened.[3] In the late nineteenth century, societal norms for middle- and upper-class women included the "cult of domesticity"—women's place was in the home. Indeed, middle- and upper-class women were considered to be in need of protection from the harsh realities of war, and they were therefore not expected to work in gruesome battlefield conditions. Instead, they were expected to stay home and do such things as knit scarves or roll bandages to be sent to the soldiers.[4] At the battlefront, convalescent soldiers assisted in the care of others who were sick or injured.

Despite the societal restrictions and the women's lack of training, within days of the firing on Fort Sumter, thousands of women from both the North and the South volunteered to serve as nurses. They did so in makeshift hospitals created from hastily converted churches, government buildings, hotels, and warehouses. In the South, where they were in closer proximity to the battlefront, some women set up hospitals in their homes.[5]

Catholic nuns were among those who volunteered to nurse, and their care was in contrast to that provided by the lady volunteers. Most upper-class lady volunteers helped by providing the soldiers with coffee, milk-punch, and other foods and necessities. They also wrote letters for the soldiers when they visited.[6] Some lay women, like Mary Ann Bickerdyke, a Union nurse who served in the West, and Phoebe Pember, who ran the Confederate Chimborazo Hospital in Richmond, Virginia, did a great deal more—organizing the camps, ordering supplies, establishing diet kitchens, and running dispensaries. For the most part, however, the women's role was confined to ancillary help. In contrast, the Catholic sisters provided direct physical care to the sick and injured. They bathed and fed the soldiers, gave medicines, and assisted with dressing changes. Some of the nuns—and a few lay women, including Catherine Lawrence, a refined, upper-class Northerner—also assisted in surgery, "tying arteries," and administering chloroform, one of the few anesthetic agents available at the time.[7]

The procedure for administering chloroform was relatively simple. The anesthetizer poured the drug over a cloth held over the patient's nose and mouth until the desired effect was achieved. However, if the anesthetist poured the chloroform too quickly, the patient would struggle violently against the feeling of suffocation. Sometimes he stopped breathing. With some experience, the Catholic sisters mastered the technique, providing invaluable assistance to the often-overwhelmed Civil War surgeons.[8]

## Post-Civil War Nursing and Medicine

In the decade after the war, formal training schools for nurses opened throughout the country—most based on the apprenticeship model advocated by Florence Nightingale in Britain.[9] Early directors of these schools emphasized general training for nurses rather than specialty education in such fields as anesthesia. Student nurses worked in operating rooms, but more often than not, they did not give anesthesia. The surgeon usually had a medical student or apprentice physician deliver the chloroform or ether, two of the most commonly used anesthetics in this era. Because the patient's initial reaction to the anesthesia was typically violent as he struggled for air, surgeons argued that the strength of a muscular male medical student was necessary to control the patient during this phase.[10]

In the years between 1865 and 1900, some Catholic sisters who had assisted in the delivery of anesthesia during the war continued to do so. Among these were Sister Mary Bernard, a nun from Wichita, Kansas, who worked at St. Vincent's Hospital in Erie, Pennsylvania in 1878; Sister Aldoza Eltrich, who administered open-drop ether and chloroform at St. John's Hospital in Springfield, Illinois in 1880; and Sister Remigus, who assisted with chloroform at Santa Rosa Infirmary in San Antonio, Texas in 1899.[11] Lay nurses who had given anesthesia during the war also continued in this role. For example, in 1887 Catherine S. Lawrence delivered anesthesia at Brooklyn Memorial Hospital in New York.[12]

During the decades following the Civil War, however, there were no formal training programs for nurse anesthetists. Some nurse training schools included a month or two of clinical experience in anesthesia delivery in the final year of coursework. Others included a smattering of theoretical content on anesthesia delivery in their classes and textbooks.[13] Nonetheless, one hospital stood out. At St. Mary's Hospital in Rochester, Minnesota, nurse-provided anesthesia would receive world recognition.[14]

In 1885, a German anesthetist visiting St. Mary's Hospital (later known as the Mayo clinic) taught Dr. William Worrall Mayo and his physician sons, Charles H. and William J., a new technique for administering anesthesia. He recommended the gradual administration of chloroform and/or ether by using a wire frame covered with gauze, which was placed over the patient's mouth and nose. The anesthetizer would slowly place drops of the anesthetic agent on the cloth until the patient lost consciousness. This method, soon labeled "the open-drop method," prevented the anesthetist from giving large quantities of the agents too rapidly.

Impressed by its effectiveness, Dr. William W. Mayo subsequently used this approach in his busy surgical practice at St. Mary's Hospital, where the Sisters of St. Francis worked. In 1889, eager to have a trained nurse assist him, Dr. Mayo hired Edith Graham, a graduate of Women's Hospital in Chicago and the only trained nurse in Rochester, to be his "anesthetist, office nurse, general bookkeeper and secretary."[15] Shortly thereafter, he taught her how to administer anesthesia using the German method.[16] Over the next four years, the Mayo team performed 655 surgical operations at St. Mary's. Of these, 98.3% were successful, in that the patients had left the hospital alive.[17] Edith Graham had given the anesthesia.

Graham continued to work as an anesthetist until 1893, when she married Dr. Charles H. Mayo. After she resigned, Graham's friend, Alice Magaw, assumed her responsibilities, again delivering anesthesia using the new "open-drop" method. Magaw was so skilled in her technique that years later Charles Mayo named her "the mother of anesthesia" for her mastery of open-drop ether administration.[18] Describing the new method, Magaw wrote:

> The inhaler used is the Esmarch mask, with two thicknesses of stockinette, and we always have both ether and chloroform ready and give whichever is indicated by the condition of the patient. In administering ether, we commence with the drop method as carefully and with as much air, as though it were chloroform, until the patient's face is flushed, when we have a large piece of surgeon's gauze of several thicknesses convenient and keep adding a few more layers of gauze and giving ether a trifle faster until the patient is asleep, then remove the gauze and continue with the same covering as at the start, and by the drop method. Should it produce difficult breathing, profuse secretion of mucus, or cough, or should the muscles be slow to relax, change to chloroform. . . . [19]

At a time when it was not unusual for a medical student to be expected to give anesthesia as he observed in the operating room, Alice Magaw challenged this tradition, asserting that the responsibility for administering anesthesia should be given to nurses instead. According to her:

> No anesthetizer can learn to be a surgeon at the same time he is administering an anesthetic, but many doctors think they will let the anesthetic take care of itself, especially in giving ether, and learn what they can at this time. When finally the attention is attracted to the patient, the result is that artificial respiration and drugs are resorted to or the patient comes out of the anesthetic when the fault has been wholly with the anesthetizer. For this reason, we think a well qualified, especially trained nurse for this purpose, can get better results, as her interests are undivided.[20]

While Magaw was advocating nurse anesthetists rather than physicians in training, a physician, Isabella Coler Herb, an 1892 graduate of Northwestern University Women's Medical School in Chicago, joined the Mayo team. Herb was to work with Charles Mayo as his anesthetist and also serve as the hospital's pathologist. She was an experienced physician. Herb had served a year-long internship at Mary Thompson Hospital for Women and Children in Chicago, where she later served as assistant to the medical staff and as dispensary physician and superintendent. Before working with the Mayo physicians, Herb also spent three and a half years as an anesthetist and pathologist at Augustana Hospital in Chicago, collaborating with Lawrence Prince, MD, a leader in the development of open-drop ether and chloroform anesthesia. In 1898, just a year before transferring to St. Mary's, Herb published her work on one thousand consecutive general anesthesia cases, the third in a series analyzing information gained from the surgeries at Augustana.[21] Because of her experience and her growing reputation, Dr. Herb was a significant addition to the Mayo team.

Five years later, in the autumn of 1904, Isabella Herb left St. Mary's Hospital for further education in Europe, and a new *nurse* anesthetist, Florence Henderson, joined the surgical group at St. Mary's Hospital.[22]

In 1905, St. Mary's opened a third operating room for Dr. E. Starr Judd, and registered nurse Mary Hines became his nurse anesthetist. In 1909, two more nurse anesthetists, Mary Shortner and Ann Powderly, also began practicing with the Mayo doctors, after receiving on-the-job training from both the surgeons and the experienced nurse anesthetists. Although that training was minimal (e.g., Ann Powderly trained with Florence Henderson for only three months before she gave anesthesia on her own), at that time it was more than anyone else had.[23]

By 1909 Henderson was clear about the limits of nursing's scope of practice in relation to anesthesia delivery. Writing in the *American Journal of Nursing,* Henderson emphasized the fact that the nurse anesthetist worked under the supervision of the surgeon. According to her: "When giving an anesthetic, a nurse must bear in mind the fact that she is still a nurse and should never anesthetize a patient unless a physician is present in the room. Neither is it within her limits to prescribe drugs."[24] Although she maintained that nurses should not prescribe anesthesia, Henderson seemed convinced that adjusting the treatment according to her skilled observations was within the legal boundaries of nursing because she worked under the direction of the surgeon.

## Necessary Knowledge for Safe Care

In the early years of the twentieth century, administering anesthesia seemed to be a simple procedure that anyone could do. In fact, there was limited scientific knowledge about the procedure and no understanding of controlled ventilation. A medical student, intern, nurse, or physician's wife, in some cases, simply put a cloth over the patient's face and dropped ether on it until the patient was asleep. Actually, the procedure was much more complicated than anyone thought, and soon a few surgeons began to realize that they could not operate unless they could trust the anesthetizer to observe the patient and keep him under the effects of the anesthetizing agent. Too much could happen. The patient could choke, tense, relax, come out of anesthesia before the surgeon completed the operation. Or the patient might experience a decrease in his respirations or pulse, or become cyanotic.[25]

Observing the patient closely was key to successful anesthesia delivery, and the surgeons recognized that trained nurse anesthetists observed the patient more closely than did medical students and interns, whose "attention was more often directed to the operation."[26] If the anesthetizer missed critical clues to the patient's condition, the patient could die. In order to monitor the patient, the anesthetist had to rely on his or her own observations, constantly observing the patient's pupils, skin color, pulse, muscle tone, and facial expression, as well as the depth and effort of respirations. According to Alice Magaw:

> The eyes give very early warning of danger. Some insist that the state of the pupils, the pulse or change in respiration are sure indications of danger, but to rely upon any one of these signs would be folly; carefully watch all of these symptoms, not relying on any one of them.[27]

Magaw and other nurse anesthetists had the skill to recognize early warning signs and symptoms because they had the necessary training to do so. They had completed anesthesia training programs after graduation from nursing school, and they specialized in the field. Discussing the importance of specialization in anesthesia, Florence Henderson wrote:

> In the nursing profession, as in all other lines of work, the tendency of the day is toward specialism, and by this means more efficient work is being accomplished. . . . By concentrating her energies she [the nurse anesthetist] will attain a degree of skill in one direction which it would impossible to acquire in all. . . . [28]

Of the few anesthesia programs available before 1900, the program at St. Mary's Hospital under the direction of the Mayo team was considered one of the best in the United States. Training there consisted of several months of apprenticeship in the practical and theoretical aspects of the work, both of which Alice Magaw and Florence Henderson considered important.[29]

By 1913 the Mayo Clinic training program was six months long. That year, Sophie Gran Jevne Winton, who would become a leader in the field of anesthesia from 1913 to her retirement in 1958, completed anesthesia training at Mayo. Twenty-one years later, in the Superior Court of California in 1934, she would be asked to testify about the nature of that education.[30]

## Documenting Safe Care

Like physician anesthesiologists Isabella Herb and Lawrence Prince, who kept records of their surgeries and published the results, nurse anesthetists kept detailed records of their work and published their outcomes in medical and nursing journals. In these articles, the nurses documented the fact that the care they gave was safe and effective. In an article published in the *St. Paul's Medical Journal*, for example, Alice Magaw reported her "Observations on 1092 Cases of Anesthesia from January 1, 1899 to January 1, 1900":

> In that time, we have administered an anesthetic 1092 times; ether alone 674 times; chloroform 245 times; ether and chloroform combined 173 times. I can report that out of this number, 1092 cases, we have not had an accident; we have not had occasion to use artificial respiration once; nor one case of ether pneumonia; neither have we had any serious renal results. Tongue forceps were used but once, the operation was on the jaw and it was quite necessary.[31]

Six years later, Alice Magaw published "A Review of Over 14000 Surgical Anesthetics" in *Surgery, Gynecology and Obstetrics,* emphasizing the fact that to decrease the need for large doses and thereby minimize complications, it was important to give the anesthetic slowly and "talk the patient to sleep."[32]

## The Art of Nurse Anesthesia

Nurse anesthetists believed there was an art to giving anesthesia and defined a gender-specific role for themselves, asserting that nurses, because they were women, were particularly suited for the job. Nurse anesthetists

Magaw and Henderson noted that a soft tone of voice and "talking the patient to sleep with as little ether as possible," was one of the benefits of having a nurse complete the anesthesia induction.[33] A few years later, Frances Truckey, a graduate of St. Vincent's Hospital Training School in Toledo, Ohio, also made mention of the unique qualities of nurse anesthetists:

> A nurse [anesthetist] of pleasing personality has a gentle, quiet way about her which makes for composure and confidence in the patient. Excitement and fear are banished by her comforting and soothing words and, in many instances, she practically sings the patient to sleep, assisted by a much smaller quantity of the anesthetic than would be possible otherwise.[34]

For years, surgeons who worked with nurse anesthetists continued this gendered line of reasoning. As Irvin D. Metzger, chairman of the State Board of Medical Education and Licensure in Harrisburg, Pennsylvania, wrote in 1936:

> It became evident, ere long experimentation, that the temperament of a woman who might be enamored by this kind of work was more suitable to its peculiar needs than that of a man; also, that her interest is more apt to be centered on her part of the care of the patient than on the entire care as is apt to be the concern of a physician-anesthetist. Some surgeons claim also that the motherly instinct of a woman exerts peculiar soothing charms over patients and makes them more amenable to drug effect . . . the consensus among recognized surgeons of this country is that with adequate training women are preferred to men in the administration of anesthetics.[35]

## Boundary Wars

Although Magaw, Henderson, and other nurses had been administering anesthesia for years, in 1911 nurse anesthetists faced the first legal challenge to their practice. That year, the New York State Medical Society declared that the administration of an anesthetic by a nurse violated state law, claiming that the nurses were practicing medicine without a license. That same year, physician anesthesiologist Isabella Herb, formerly of the Mayo Clinic, broke with the Mayo physicians' support of nurse anesthetists and published an article in the *Journal of the American Medical Association*, taking a stance against any anesthetizer who was not a physician.

As an experienced physician anesthetist, Isabella Herb was determined to provide "the highest quality of anesthesia."[36] She was also interested in advancing the science of anesthesiology and developing anesthesia as a medical rather than a nursing specialty. Her arguments never included the possibility that nurse anesthetists created an economic threat to physician anesthetists. She had plenty of work. In fact, physician anesthetists were a rare breed. Herb herself invoked a gendered role for women, but in her case it was women *physician* anesthetists who had the advantage of possessing the soft voice and gentle manner that surgeons valued. Furthermore, women *physician* anesthetists had the scientific knowledge that physicians gained in medical school. Dr. Herb was not against nurse anesthetists because of their incompetence or lack of skill. In fact, she respected the nurses' abilities, but she established a clear boundary between nursing and medicine. What Herb was concerned about was the advancement of the scientific knowledge about anesthesia. According to her:

> Nurses, when properly trained, make very good anesthetizers, but . . . because of their lack of medical training, they are unable to weigh physical findings and . . . are unable to decide which anesthetic is safest. Therefore, no hope of advancement or research work [in the field of anesthesia] can be expected.[37]

Dr. Herb had a valid concern—nurses in the early decades of the twentieth century did not have in-depth knowledge of anatomy and physiology, pathology, chemistry, or other basic sciences. In addition, they did not conduct independent research to advance the science. Herb was also aware that the Mayo's use of nurse anesthetists was an anomaly. Throughout the country, most surgeons used medical students or interns, whom Herb labeled "persons with absolutely no training,"[38] to assist with anesthesia.

Isabella Herb's influence soon spread. She based her observations and anesthesia techniques on scientific facts. In addition, she was articulate and well published. Furthermore, her explanations about the effects of anesthesia were more thorough than the nurses' discussion of the same topic, and they were also based on the science available at the time. For example, explaining the effects of administering too much chloroform, Herb wrote:

> In chloroform toxemia, the arterial tension is so lowered that the blood supply to the respiratory center is reduced and breathing fails from this cause as much as from the sedative action of the anesthetic. Death may also be due to asphyxia, as in administering nitrous-oxide with an insufficient amount of oxygen.[39]

In contrast, nurse anesthetist Alice Magaw based her recommendations for dealing with the same phenomenon on her professional experience of the patient's reactions rather than on the underlying science. Writing in 1900, Magaw noted: "Chloroform should be given with more air, and in less quantity and with the regular drop [method] instead of the stream as so many use. . . . It should be given slowly and carefully as it acts very quickly."[40] Both Herb's and Magaw's explanations were correct and useful in that they both recommended the careful administration of the agent with sufficient air/oxygen. Herb's explanation, however, was clearly more scholarly than Magaw's.

Isabella Herb's publications also reflected her concern that the field of anesthesia was becoming more complicated as new anesthetic agents were discovered and put to use. As she noted in a paper read before the Third Annual Meeting of the American Association of Anesthetists in San Francisco on June 21, 1915—with the introduction of ether, giving anesthesia would not be as simple a technique as it had been in the past. In fact, in the future, chloroform might not be used. According to Herb: "With modern appliances for the administration of ether by vaporization, the field of usefulness for chloroform has been very materially lessened."[41]

Herb was not alone in her concern for advancement in the growing medical specialty of anesthesia. The next year, the members of the Interstate Association of Anesthetists elected her as chairman at their July 1916 meeting in Louisville, Kentucky.[42] There, the physicians "unanimously resolved that the Association through its officers, its official journal and its individual members bring to a definite conclusion the administration of anesthetics by unlicensed [in medicine] persons in every state."[43]

Not all physicians supported the resolution. Only the year before, in 1915, Dr. George W. Crile had established The Lakeside Hospital School of Anesthesia in Cleveland, Ohio, in cooperation with nurse anesthetist Agatha Hodgins, for the purpose of training nurse anesthetists. Now, in 1916, when the physician's association passed the resolution, Crile was not about to close the school. As a result, the state's medical society brought a lawsuit against the Lakeside program on the grounds that the nurse anesthetists were practicing medicine when they administered anesthesia and made adjustments in the dose. Despite their efforts, the medical society lost the case, and the amended Ohio state medical practice act subsequently protected the practice of nurse anesthesia.

After that legal decision, the physicians continued their opposition. In 1917, Kentucky's Jefferson County Medical Society sued Dr. Lewis Frank for having nurse anesthetist Margaret Hatfield deliver anesthesia to his patients (*Frank v. South*). Once again, the medical society argued that the

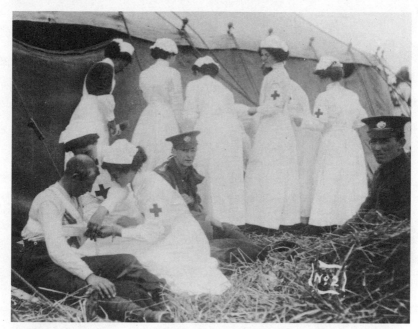

Figure 2.1: Red Cross nurses, World War I. KC, CNHI

nurse anesthetist's independent assessments of the patient's condition during surgery and her subsequent adjustments in the doses and types of anesthetics were equivalent to the acts of diagnosis and prescription. According to the physicians' logic, Hatfield was illegally practicing medicine.

Once again, the case went to court and once again, the physicians lost the case, even after appeal. In fact, the Kentucky appellate court ruled that anesthesia provided by nurse anesthetist Margaret Hatfield did not constitute the practice of medicine if it was given under the orders and supervision of a licensed physician (Dr. Louis Frank).[44] In essence, the court declared nurse anesthesia legal but "subordinate" to the medical profession. The underlying question, of course, was whether or not Margaret Hatfield was prescribing a drug when she gave anesthesia, or whether she was simply administering a drug under the supervision and direction of the surgeon.

Meanwhile, throughout the United States, numerous schools of anesthesia opened between 1912 and 1920, each offering six months of postgraduate nursing education in the specialty. Included among these schools were Johns Hopkins, Barnes, New York Hospital, and Presbyterian Hospital in Chicago.[45] By mid-decade, some of these hospital programs were preparing army nurses to administer ether and chloroform to casualties of battle. In 1914 Europe was already at war, and American nurses were volunteering to serve with the British and French nurses already at the front.

## World War I: New Opportunities for Nurse Anesthetists

By the time the United States entered World War I in 1917, the specialty of nurse anesthesia was fairly well established. Based on an interesting and unique set of circumstances, it had also been decided that nurse anesthetists would be used at the European front in the American Base Hospitals.

Despite President Woodrow Wilson's commitment to neutrality, both he and the Congress had made preparations for the United States's involvement in the European war, should it become necessary. In 1916, Dr. William J. Mayo had been named chairman of the Committee of American Physicians for Medical Preparedness (later renamed the General Medical Board of the Council for the Defense after the United States declared war). His brother, Dr. Charles H. Mayo, was named a member. The committee also recruited other physicians into a medical reserve corps. One of these doctors was Dr. George Crile from Lakeside Hospital, who initiated a plan to organize 50 base hospitals that would be held in readiness as Red Cross hospitals—converted to military hospitals should the need arise. Each base hospital would be located 50 miles behind the front line of battle; have 500 beds; and be staffed by 27 medical officers, 60 nurses, and 153 enlisted men. Staff, funds, and supplies would be donated by large hospitals and medical schools.[46]

Crile's plan also called for the use of nurse anesthetists. Both he and the Mayo physicians had worked with nurse anesthetists for over a decade and admired their work. In fact, Crile had recently opened the Lakeside Program. Thus, including nurse anesthetists in the plans for staffing the base hospitals was an obvious answer to the question of who would administer anesthesia to the wounded soldiers.

## Base Hospital #26: The Mayo Unit

Early in the war effort, the surgeon general had selected the Mayo Clinic to sponsor the base hospital from Minnesota. Dr. William Mayo thought it more appropriate, however, that the medical school of the University of Minnesota sponsor the base hospital and delegated the job to Dr. Arthur Law, associate professor of surgery at the university. Law began to organize Base Hospital #26 in the spring of 1917, and the Mayo brothers, committed to doing all they could, contributed $15,000 of its $30,000 fundraising goal. Their contribution was essentially one-quarter of the $60,000 total raised by the American Red Cross, private citizens, the University of Minnesota, and others—a substantial sum. Because of the

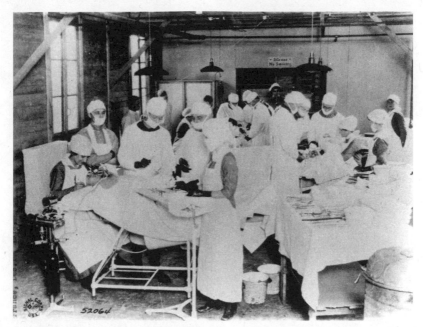

Figure 2.2: World War I military operating room, France. AANA HF

doctors' generous financial support, Base Hospital #26 was able to purchase state-of-the-art equipment and supplies. In addition, five nurses
from the Mayo Clinic volunteered to go overseas with the group. Among
them was Nell Bryant, the only one trained as a nurse anesthetist.[47] Her
story serves as an example of the work the nurse anesthetists did.

Bryant immediately received orders from the war department to go to
Lakewood, New Jersey. On April 17, 1918 she was transferred to the Nurses'
Mobilization Station at the Holley Hotel in New York City, where she prepared for her war duties by learning military protocols and being fitted for
uniforms. Shortly thereafter, on June 4 the army nurses embarked on their
trans-Atlantic crossing, arriving in Liverpool, England on June 16, 1918.
From there, Bryant traveled to the French Village of Allerey to Base Hospital
#26, one of ten base hospitals in a large camp. The first to be completed,
Base Hospital #26 was designated the surgical hospital (while others were
labeled the "contagious, venereal disease, eye, mental" etc.). Because of its
leadership and its staff, Base Hospital #26 was also called "the Mayo Unit."[48]

Bryant did not stay long in Allerey, but went almost immediately to
Mobile Hospital No.1—at the front line of combat, about three hours by
train from Paris. The mobile hospital had eighteen operating tables and
eighteen surgical teams, all kept busy when the wounded arrived directly
from the trenches of Château-Thierry, an area of significant fighting.[49]

The realities of the Front were gruesome—shrapnel created devastating wounds, and mustard gas destroyed lungs and caused profound burns. The resulting need for pain relief and anesthesia care for the wounded soldiers created an immediate demand for anesthetists. Nurse anesthetists not only had the knowledge and skills necessary to meet that demand, but they could also relieve hundreds of doctors for medical and surgical work.[50] Another Mayo Clinic graduate, Sophie Winton, working at Mobile Hospital No. 1 during the battle of Château-Thierry, described the demands on the surgeons and her own responsibilities:

> During the drives, patients came in so fast that all the surgeons could do was to remove bullets and shrapnel, stop hemorrhages, and put iodoform packs in the wounds and bandage them. As soon as they were through operating on one patient, I would have to have the next patient anesthetized.[51]

## Anesthesia in the War

At the battlefront, physician and nurse anesthetists used both ether and chloroform as the anesthetic agents of choice. Dr. George Crile, the founder of the Lakeside School in Cleveland and the originator of the base hospital plan, toured the camps to investigate the surgeon's needs. On one trip, he took along a supply of nitrous oxide-oxygen, inhalation agents on which he and Agatha Hodgins had been experimenting in Ohio for patients in shock. Crile's intent was to use them at the front. However, he soon found that these compressed gases were too cumbersome, expensive, and explosive to be used anywhere near the battle.[52] Instead, it became apparent that ether should be used. In contrast to the explosive inhalation agents, ether could be readily delivered to wounded soldiers via the open-drop method for which the Mayo Clinic anesthetists were renowned.[53]

Using ether was the simple solution, but at the front nothing was simple. The ether available in Europe was of poor quality, and was bulky and explosive. It also caused the patient to cough and to produce copious amounts of mucus that could exacerbate the incidence of postoperative pneumonia. Clearly, "old-fashioned" chloroform was more practical,[54] at least for the initial induction. According to a 1916 article in the *American Journal of Surgery Anesthesia Supplement*:

> Chloroform, owing to its efficiency, compactness and ease of transportation, retains its erstwhile superiority as the anesthetic of war.

The bulk and explosiveness of ether renders it less desirable as a routine agent.[55]

Hence, the Americans used chloroform for induction, then ether to maintain the anesthetic state.[56] And once again, it became apparent that nurse anesthetists were skilled at the administration of chloroform.

Recognizing the growing need for more nurse anesthetists, the army sent twenty nurses to the Mayo Clinic to study the art and science of anesthesia. Their program was only six weeks long—only a fraction of the length of the usual training.[57] The army nurses were needed back in Europe as soon as possible. According to historian Mary Sarnecky:

> During the first week in Minnesota, the Army nurses merely observed the activities of a regular anesthetist in the operating room. They then gradually assumed the anesthetist's responsibilities. . . . [T]he students continued doing more until they had total charge of the patient's anesthesia. . . . The goal was to have the Army nurses administer anesthesia to fifty patients . . . on her own . . . before she left.[58]

The training period had been shortened from six months to six weeks. Nevertheless, the nurse was required to demonstrate competence in anesthesia delivery prior to going to the front.

## The 1920s: Developing the Science

During World War I, nurse anesthesia had made its mark. The following decade was one of continued progress for the nurses, as well as one in which resistance to the nurse anesthetist role grew behind the scenes. The progress was remarkable. Surgeons all over the country were using nurse anesthetists. The trend even extended to university hospitals. In 1922, nurse anesthetist Alice M. Hunt responded to a request from Dr. Samuel Harvey, a Yale professor of surgery, to "send me a nurse anesthetist," by accepting the offer herself. The offer included her appointment as an instructor of anesthesia with university rank at the Yale Medical School, a significant and prestigious appointment for a nurse.[59]

Although Hunt was employed by a university, nurse anesthetists were more frequently hired by nursing departments in small-town hospitals. For example, Florence A. McQuillen, who would later serve as the executive director of the American Association of Nurse Anesthetists, was offered a position as superintendent of nurses in a small hospital in Glasgow,

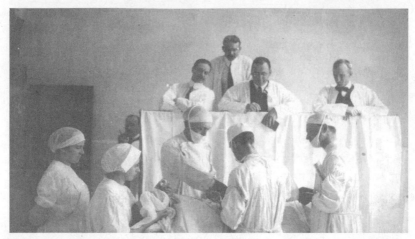

Figure 2.3: St. Mary's Hospital Operating Room, circa 1920s. AANA Archives 94–190

Montana. She was expected to give ether as part of her job, even though she had had only two months of experience in anesthesia delivery during her final year of nurses' training.[60]

Not only were the nurse anesthetists getting job offers, they were also gaining legal status. The revised Ohio Medical Practice Act, Section 1286-2, effective August 2, 1927, allowed nurses to give anesthesia. According to that statute:

> Nothing in this chapter shall be construed to apply to or prohibit in any way, the administration of an anesthetic by a registered nurse under the direction of and in the immediate presence of a licensed physician, provided such nurse has taken a prescribed course in anesthesia, at a hospital in good standing.[61]

The conditions were of course, that the nurse worked under the supervision of a physician.

The problem was that physicians themselves wanted to practice anesthesia. In fact, during the 1920s, as surgeries increased in number in hospitals across the nation and new scientific findings emerged, more physicians began to choose anesthesia as their specialty. With the discovery of new anesthetic agents like ethyl chloride, the science of anesthesia was indeed evolving at a rapid pace, and as a result, the field was becoming more interesting to physicians. After Dr. Arthur Guedel, a 1908 graduate of the Medical College of Indiana who had served as an anesthesiologist in France during the war, published his seminal work on the signs and stages of ether anesthesia,[62] the field had even more appeal. Physician anesthesia training programs increased in length, and possibilities for research in the field expanded. Physician anesthetists were also forming professional groups. One of these, the Pacific Coast Association of [MD] Anesthetists, formed in 1922 and immediately incorporated into the California Medical Society,[63] would later play a significant role in challenging the right of nurses to practice in this field.

Meanwhile, six years after its formation, the California Medical Society was actively trying to restrict nurses from the field of anesthesia. In March 1928, the California Board of Medical Examiners adopted a resolution and sent it to all hospitals in California, requesting the termination of nurse anesthetists on the grounds that they were practicing in violation of the state's medical practice act.[64] Part of the physicians' concern was financial. The fee for nurse anesthetists was absorbed into the cost of the surgery, so using them appeared to more economical. Physician anesthesiologists billed separately, and doctors often used anesthesia administration as a way to supplement their incomes.[65] By 1929, with the stock market crash and the subsequent devastation of the American economy, their income from anesthesia work would no longer be supplemental. In fact, during what would later be called "The Great Depression," physicians needed work as much as the nurses did, and nurse anesthetists soon were regarded as a threat to physicians' incomes.

## The 1930s: The Depression Years

During the early 1930s, the country was in the throes of a severe economic depression, and jobs were scarce. As many physicians found their medical practice less remunerative because their patients could not afford to pay, they tried "to restore to themselves" the field of anesthesia practice.[66] And, with the devastation of the American economy, tension increased between nurse anesthetists and physicians. Meanwhile, during this time the science of anesthesia grew at an exponential rate. New drugs were being discovered, and experimentation was underway. Two of the most important innovations were the introduction of the new agent cyclopropane and the development of intratracheal anesthesia.[67] Physicians were definitely interested. Thus, the stage was set for increasing conflict between the two groups: physicians wanted work in the developing specialty, and nurse anesthetists, supported by the American Hospital Association, continued to give most of the anesthesia administered in hospitals across America.

At the same time, nurse anesthetists were organizing. In 1931, Agatha Hodgins established the National Association of Nurse Anesthetists (later to become the American Association of Nurse Anesthetists, or the AANA). Its principal aims were "to promote the science and art of anesthesiology and to do all things necessary to achieve protection to the patient and the public in the administration of anesthetics."[68] At the first annual meeting of the organization, held in 1933 in Milwaukee, Wisconsin, Dr. Bert W. Caldwell, executive secretary of the American Hospital Association (AHA), noted that "2,000 institutions in the U.S. were employing the services of nurse anesthetists."[69]

Recognizing that although they had the numbers, nurse anesthetists still needed affiliation with a larger nursing organization if they were to successfully lobby for the right to practice, the National Association of Nurse Anesthetists voted to affiliate with the American Nurses Association (ANA). Despite their intentions to gain the support of the nurses' association, the nurse anesthetists were not successful. In fact, the ANA, afraid to assume legal responsibility for a group that could be charged with practicing medicine without a license, refused to include nurse anesthetists.[70]

Thus, by 1934, when the Los Angeles County Medical Association, represented by William Chalmers-Francis, sued Dagmar Nelson for "the illegal practice of medicine, in violation of the Medical Practice Act"[71] (as noted in the opening section of this chapter), nurse anesthetists were facing resistance from both the nursing and the medical professions. Nelson, formerly a nurse anesthetist at the Mayo Clinic, had moved to California with her husband several years earlier and had been delivering anesthesia unopposed until this lawsuit. The trial, which began on July 12, 1934, lasted twelve days. For the entire session, nurse anesthetist Sophie Winton (who had also trained at Mayo) was present in the courtroom, at one time testifying about her work as a nurse anesthetist and the training she had received.[72] In the end, the Honorable Allen B. Campbell (the judge), decided in favor of Nelson, concluding that:

> The administration of general anesthetics by the defendant Dagmar
> A. Nelson, pursuant to the directions and supervision of duly
> licensed physicians and surgeons, as shown by the evidence in this
> case, does not constitute the practice of medicine or surgery, within
> the meaning of the laws of the State of California, and . . . constitutes the practice of nursing within the meaning of the laws of the
> State of California.[73]

Clearly, the nurses had won the case. In response, William Chalmers-Frances, MD, filed another suit against Nelson in 1936, which again resulted in a favorable judgment for nursing.[74] In 1938, however, that ruling was appealed to the California Supreme Court. This time, when the

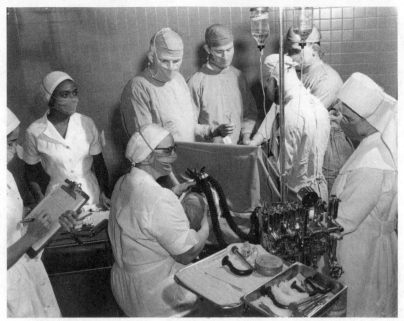

Figure 2.4: Helen Lamb (seated). Barnes Hospital, St. Louis, circa 1940s. AANA HF.

case was heard, the *amicus curiae* brief submitted by the National Association of Nurse Anesthetists (NANA) argued that the reason for this lawsuit was primarily economic, resulting from the severe depression that had affected the entire country. As the NANA lawyer noted in the introduction to the brief:

> Since the onset of the economic disturbance of the past few years, agitation has sprung up in certain quarters to restrict the right to administer anesthetics to . . . licensed physicians, thus eliminating nurse anesthetists from the field of anesthesia. We believe that the aforesaid economic disturbance and the agitation against the nurse anesthetist bear a direct relationship.[75]

The National Association of Nurse Anesthetists also argued that the "safety of the patient is the most important thing to be considered in determining whether a nurse anesthetist ought to be permitted to administer anesthetics" and that "the nurse anesthetist is content to rest her case with surgeons and laymen alike on that single proposition."[76] The court again ruled in favor of Nelson, stating that she was not practicing medicine because she was "under the immediate direction and supervision of the operating surgeon."[77] As of 1938, legal precedent had been established three times; the administration of anesthesia by a nurse was within the scope of nursing practice. The ruling was based on the premise that nurses were not prescribing, that in fact, the operating physician took responsibility for prescribing the anesthetic in the first place.

Although the legal precedent was positive for nursing, the courts, the physicians who supported the practice of nurse anesthesia, the medical and nursing associations, and the nurse anesthetists themselves all skirted the real issues: (1) were nurse anesthetists competent to prescribe? and (2) who controlled the practice of nursing—medicine or nursing? These two issues would continue to be topics of contention in other places and for nurses working in other expanded roles throughout the remainder of the century. What would become increasingly clear was the fact that when the nurses were not an economic threat to physicians—when they worked in undesirable locations or with minority populations—they were considered competent to do whatever needed to be done. Moreover, as long as the medical profession supervised nursing practice and organized medicine did not challenge the expanded role, nurses could take on tasks formerly done by physicians.

CHAPTER 3

# Providing Care in the "Hoot Owl Hollers"

## Nursing, Medicine, and the Law in the Frontier Nursing Service, 1925–1950

See we nurses don't prescribe and we don't diagnose. We can make a tentative diagnosis and we can give that to the doctor, and if there's anything wrong then he'll tell us how to treat it. So they [the doctors] gave us this Routine of things that we could use and the things we could do——and the things we couldn't do.

Betty Lester, RN[1]

During an oral interview in 1978, Betty Lester, a certified nurse-midwife, reflected on her work as assistant field supervisor in the Frontier Nursing Service (FNS) in the early 1920s and 1930s. In those years, Lester had had unprecedented freedom to manage patients in the remote, mountainous region of Leslie County, Kentucky. Recounting that experience years later, Lester denied the extent of the freedom she had actually had. Like other registered nurses in the first half of the twentieth century, Lester had been socialized to defer to physicians' judgment and orders. So, when recalling her experiences in the FNS later in her life, Lester did not take ownership of the clinical decision-making process she had used. Instead, Lester acknowledged only that she and other Frontier nurses made "tentative diagnoses," reporting those to a physician associated with the FNS. In reality, she had often practiced on her own, as there were few phones in the isolated community during the 1920s and 1930s, and physicians were rarely available to consult in person. In contrast to Lester's perceptions, for all practical purposes, the diagnoses made by the FNS nurses were the only diagnoses, and their treatment was the only treatment.

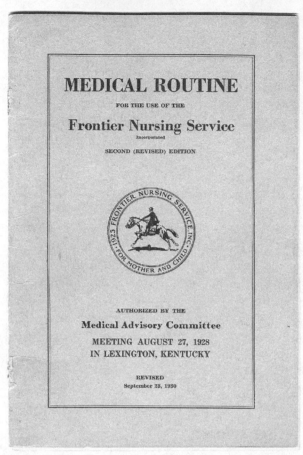

Figure 3.1: *Medical Routine Revised 1930.* UK-SC, 85MI, box 27, folder 2

The "Routines" to which Lester referred were physicians' standing orders that legally covered the nurses' actions.[2] Because of these, no one ever questioned the nurses' practice among the isolated highland people.[3] In their correspondence with Mary Breckenridge, the founder of the FNS, it is quite clear that several of the doctors who practiced in the Appalachian community had a collegial relationship with the nurses and trusted both Mary Breckenridge's expertise and the nurses' judgment.[4] Moreover, in each of the editions of the *Medical Routines,* the physicians recognized that without the FNS nurses, the inhabitants of Leslie County would not receive care.[5] Indeed, just as the Henry Street visiting nurses provided access to care for poverty-stricken immigrants in New York City, the Frontier Nursing Service provided access to medical and nursing care for numerous poverty-stricken Scots-Irish, English, and Welsh descendants in the extreme southeastern section of Kentucky.

## Origins of the Frontier Nursing Service

For decades, attracting physicians to the remote mountainous area of Kentucky, twenty-four miles from Hazard, the nearest town, had been practically impossible. Leslie County, an area of 373 square miles with a population of fewer than 11,000, was one of the poorest and most inaccessible areas in the United States.[6] The few doctors who worked there resided in small towns some distance from the highlanders, who lived in the hollows and on the branches and headwaters of the creeks that wound through the valleys of the mountain belt.[7]

Since the early 1900s, Leslie County had also had one of the highest maternal and infant mortality rates in the United States, 124.0 deaths per 10,000 live births—whereas the national maternal death rate was 7.0 per 1,000 live births in 1929. (This rate was almost double that in England and Wales, where maternal mortality was 4.3 per 1,000 live births.)[8] Faced with this unacceptable situation, the Kentucky State Board of Health formed the Bureau of Maternal and Child Health in 1922 and charged it with the protection and promotion of the health of mothers and children in the state. Kentucky physicians, long aware of the problem, took a particular interest in addressing it.[9]

Mary Breckenridge, a member of a distinguished and well-connected Kentucky family,[10] was also interested in the problem. Breckenridge, a graduate of St. Luke's Hospital School of Nursing, had lost two children to childhood diseases; as a result, she resolved to improve maternal and child care in the United States. After obtaining training in Public Health Nursing in Boston, serving in World War I as director of child hygiene and public health nursing from 1919 to 1922, and then studying public health at Teachers College in New York City, Breckenridge went to Appalachia to work with Dr. Arthur McCormack, the state health officer for Kentucky. Once there, Breckenridge traveled the area on horseback, studying the state of obstetrical services in three mountain counties. She found that most of the highland women used uneducated, elderly Anglo-Saxon midwives to attend their babies' births, and that the untrained midwives' care was inconsistent and often of poor quality owing to practices based on superstition rather than fact.[11] According to Breckenridge:

> When I asked those of more limited practice what they would do if they had certain complication to meet I found that rarely had they decided beforehand on a plan of action. "Never had hit happen yit," [sic] was the usual answer and with it they appeared satisfied. . . . Of all obstetrical complications a hemorrhage was the most frequent . . . concerning which there seemed to be the greatest variety of supersti-

tious practices . . . [including] cording the leg . . . putting an ax
under the bed . . . and using "black gum bark from the north side of
a tree mixed with the bark of a sweet apple tree."[12]

Breckenridge also found that the distances and road conditions in the
highland region were formidable, making it almost impossible for patients
to access the few state-licensed physicians who worked in nearby towns.[13]

Given these conditions, Breckenridge concluded that the creation of a
decentralized nurse-midwifery service would be necessary to reach the
mountain people and provide them with a higher quality of care. She soon
set about preparing herself to establish this service. After obtaining midwifery training at the British Hospital for Mothers and Babies in London
to qualify herself to see patients, and seeing for herself the effectiveness of
nurse-midwives in the Scottish Highlands, Breckinridge returned to Leslie
County in 1925 and founded the Frontier Nursing Service, intending to
showcase nurse-midwives.[14] Using her extensive family and political connections for both fund raising and political support, Breckenridge
engaged members of the Appalachian community to help build
Wendover, the log house that would serve as the main headquarters for the
FNS in Hyden (population 300).[15] The house overlooked Hurricane
Creek, a wide, shallow stream that the nurses used in the absence of roads
as a route of transportation to reach the hollows.

Over the next ten years, Breckenridge established the decentralized
services she had envisioned. Frontier Nursing Service nurses worked out
of eight clinics: the main one at Wendover, Beech Fork, Red Bird, Flat
Creek, Brutus, Oneida, Bob Fork, and Wooton. All these clinics were
accessible by creek beds. Serving families in three counties altogether, each
clinic provided services to an area covering seventy-eight square miles of
the rugged Appalachian territory.[16]

## National and State Initiatives

Breckenridge's project coincided with the national initiative to provide
medical and nursing services to mothers and babies in an attempt to
decrease overall maternal and infant mortality in the United States. In
1912, in response to high national infant and maternal mortality rates and
other social problems pertaining to children, President William Howard
Taft created a federal Children's Bureau and charged it with investigating
and reporting on "all matters pertaining to the welfare of children and
child life among all classes of people."[17] The Bureau's first assignment was
to study why so many American infants died. Part of this investigation led

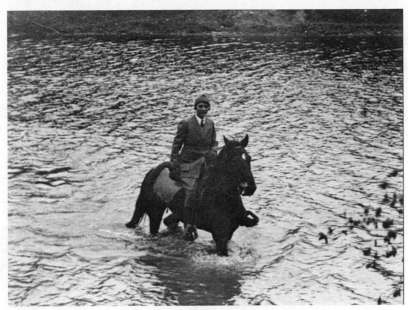

Figure 3.2: FNS nurse on horseback crossing creek.  Caufield & Shook Collection, Ekstrom Library, University of Louisville

to a national discussion of issues related to lay midwife licensing and control, as well as the question of the safety of their practice. Of concern was the lack of prenatal services provided by lay midwives, inconsistencies in their hygienic practices and their level of competence, and particularly their lack of formal training. One solution, proposed by Chicago physician Frederick J. Taussig at a 1914 meeting of the National Organization of Public Health Nurses, was that the creation of nurse-midwives rather than granny midwives might solve the "midwife question."[18] In that speech, Taussig recommended that nurse-midwifery schools be established to train graduate nurses in midwifery skills.[19] Later in the decade, under Director Julia Lathrop, the Children's Bureau recommended that public health nurses teach principles of hygiene and prenatal care to the granny midwives.[20] Then, in 1921, Congress passed the Sheppard Towner Maternity and Infant Protection Act, appropriating federal financial aid to each state ($10,000 in matching funds) for "the purpose of reducing the maternal and infant mortality and protecting the health of mothers and infants."[21] Indeed, maternal and infant mortality had the nation's attention.

In fact, the concern for safe deliveries and the public's growing acceptance of hospitals led to a decline in the use of lay midwives for deliveries. During the 1920s increasing numbers of upper- and middle-class urban white women began to use obstetricians to deliver their babies in hospitals.[22]

In contrast, poor, urban European immigrants, like those on the Lower East Side of New York City, continued to turn to midwives and continued to deliver their babies at home. Likewise, in rural southern states like Mississippi, where half the population was black, the majority of women continued to rely on African American granny midwives to deliver their babies.[23] In Leslie County, Kentucky, most women turned to untrained Anglo-Saxon granny midwives, many of whom were illiterate, to attend their babies' births. As one woman recalled: "The granny woman just came and done what she could—and she hardly ever come back. . . . Back before the [FNS] nurses came, that's all they had—just them old women."[24] It was increasingly clear: physician-assisted, hospital births were for patients of higher socioeconomic status; lay midwives attended the poor. In Leslie County, the result was high maternal and infant mortality.

Mindful of this problem, the Kentucky State Board of Health formed the Bureau of Maternal and Child Health in 1922 and charged it with the protection and promotion of the health of mothers and children in the state. Kentucky physicians, long aware of the problem of high maternal and infant mortality statistics, took a "particular interest" in addressing the matter. In 1926, the state medical society and the Louisville Obstetrical Society requested a "thorough study of every maternal death," after which they concluded that every pregnant woman should place herself "under the care of a competent physician at once."[25]

The recommendation was unrealistic. In fact, in Leslie County there were only five "state-registered physicians who could see patients and all of them (with the exception of one employed by the mission settlement school) charged $1.00 per mile for every mile spent in travel to the case, as well as an additional basic charge of $5.00."[26] Needless to say, families with an average income of $183.53 a year could not afford these prices. Moreover, the treacherous mountain terrain and the lack of roads and bridges made access to physicians difficult, even for those who could afford the fees. According to one report:

> In most instances, there is no telephone service available, some one
> must ride the entire distance, varying from 4 to 20 miles, to summon
> the doctor, who usually lives in some small village or town where he
> maintains a practice. It is often impossible for him to leave his patients
> for the length of time necessary to make a trip into the mountains. . . .
> If time and weather conditions permit, they will in an emergency visit
> those on the outskirts of their own territory. . . . In winter, when snow
> covers the ground and the creek beds are frozen, it is difficult if not
> impossible for the mountaineer to go for the doctor and equally out of
> the question for the doctor to come to the patient.[27]

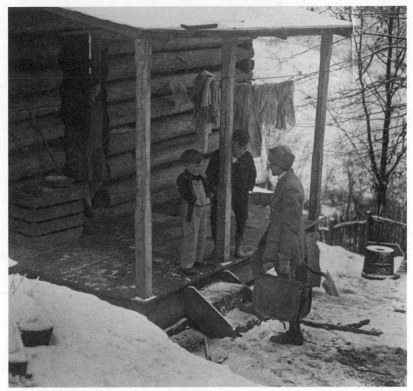

Figure 3.3: FNS nurse visiting home. FNSC, CNHI

The physician shortage in Kentucky, the difficulties of the mountainous terrain, and the national and state campaigns to reduce maternal and infant mortality, coupled with growing concerns about lay midwives, all influenced local physicians to consider the idea that using nurse-midwives might be a solution. In fact, by 1925, when Breckenridge introduced the idea of a nurse-run service, the medical community was ready to support it. Besides, Breckenridge arranged to pay half of the salary ($1,500.00) for Dr. Capps, the health officer of Leslie County, so that he would serve as "general consultant" to the nurses and treat any patients they admitted to the hospital in the small town of Hyden, only a few miles from Wendover.[28]

## Assuring Physician Supervision and Collaboration

Breckenridge was careful to observe the law in establishing the FNS, stating: "the nurse-midwives [originally British nurse-midwives and American public health nurses whom she had sent to England for midwifery train-ing[29]] were to work under supervision, [in] compliance with the regula-tions for midwives of the State Board of Health and the law governing the registration of nurses, and in cooperation with the nearest medical serv-ice."[30] The legal climate in Kentucky, particularly the statutes governing the practice of nursing during the first half of the twentieth century, sup-ported Breckenridge's ideas. A decade earlier, the Kentucky Act of 1914 had established a State Board of Examiners of Trained Nurses and required all nurses in Kentucky to be registered. The law further dictated that all applicants

> furnish satisfactory evidence that he or she is at least 21 years of age, of good moral character and has been graduated from a school for nurses . . . approved by the board. . . . Such person shall be required to undergo an examination . . . and shall pass the same to the satis-faction of the majority of said board.[31]

Nowhere did the 1914 Kentucky law specify exactly what the practice of nursing encompassed. In fact, like many of the original registration acts passed by other states, from their inception until 1955, the Kentucky laws regulating nursing practice were vague. As historian Bonnie Bullough argued: "None of the original registration acts included a definition of nursing in terms of the scope of professional practice; thus these acts are more accurately called nurse *registration* acts rather than nurse *practice* acts."[32]

Federal drug laws, equally unclear with regard to the practice of nurs-ing, also supported Breckenridge's vision for a nurse-run service. In 1914, the United States Congress had enacted the Harrison Narcotic Act, limit-ing the amount of morphine, heroin, and opium in over-the-counter remedies and reinforcing the fact that physicians, dentists, and veterinary surgeons could dispense and distribute "the aforesaid drugs only within the practice of their professional duties."[33] Nowhere in the narcotic act was the nurse's role with regard to narcotics specifically delineated. Relevant to the Frontier Nurses' work, the law did *not* restrict nurses from carrying narcotics in their bags, nor did it prohibit them from administering nar-cotics according to physicians' standing orders.

Another law, regulating the practice of nurse anesthesia (as noted in chapter 2), also helped lay the groundwork for the Frontier Nursing Service. In 1917, almost a decade prior to Breckenridge's work in Appalachia, Kentucky had been the scene of the interprofessional conflict between the Jefferson County Medical Society and Dr. Lewis Frank. In fact, the society had sued Frank for having his nurse anesthetist deliver anesthesia. The case was decided in favor of Frank and the nurse anesthetist, however. In the landmark decision of *Frank v. South,* the Kentucky appellate court ruled that anesthesia provided by nurse anesthetist Margaret Hatfield did not constitute the practice of medicine *if it was given under the orders and supervision of a licensed physician.* Of particular importance to the Frontier Nursing Service in the 1920s, in that decision the court had also noted:

> The usual practice, in this state, in cases where graduate or trained nurses are in attendance, has been for such nurses to administer hypodermics of morphia, atropia, ergo, and other drugs, when same were directed to be given by the physician in charge, in definite doses and at definite intervals, and frequently such is done by the nurses in the absence of the physician, but in accordance with his directions. . . . [34]

In order to comply with Kentucky law, Breckenridge had to do only one thing—set up an advisory committee of physicians who would write "directions" for the FNS nurses, be available for consultation, and accept referrals. In this mission Breckenridge was particularly fortunate, as her family had numerous political connections in the area. In addition, Mary Breckenridge had a cousin, Scott Breckenridge, MD, who practiced medicine in Lexington. She was also a close friend of Josephine Hunt, MD, who also practiced in the area. In 1925, Breckenridge appointed both of these doctors to the Kentucky Committee for Mothers and Babies, the same committee that three years later would become the medical advisory committee to the Frontier Nursing Service. The 1928 committee would include not only Scott Breckenridge and Josephine Hunt, but also seven other physicians,[35] all of whom were located in Lexington, about 165 miles from Wendover. Despite the distance, these physicians supervised the FNS nurses in delivering not only midwifery services, but also in providing essential medical care. Sometimes contact was made by telephone; more frequently, consultation was requested and provided through handwritten notes carried by a messenger. In most instances, however, the nurses saw patients on their own. To cover the nurses' actions in those situations, the doctors wrote "standing orders"—called *Routines* or *Medical Routines*—for the nurses to follow in their absence. In the preface to the 1928 manual, the physicians acknowledged the realities of the nurses' practice, recognizing that they worked "under extremely difficult conditions in very remote areas . . . in many instances when physicians can never be had, owing to impossible seasons of ice and 'tides,' as well as great distances and heavy mileage costs."[36] Because there were few roads in the remote Appalachian region, the nurses traveled by horseback along creek beds and mountain

trails to attend births and care for the sick, carrying their manuals every-
where. Writing in the *American Journal of Nursing* in 1938, British nurse-
midwife Vanda Summers recounted how the FNS nurses worked:

> The whole of the district work of the FNS in the Kentucky moun-
> tains is done with the aid of two pairs of saddle-bags. . . . In these
> bags we have everything needed for a home delivery. . . . In one of
> the pockets we carry our *Medical Routines* which tells us what we
> may—and may not—do. . . . [37]

Another FNS nurse commented on the contents of the saddle-bags,
noting:

> The delivery bags were set aside for delivery . . . the general bags had
> medicines in them of all sorts. And ointments and things . . . enough
> that you could give them out to people along the way if you were
> either called into a house or stopped on the road. . . . We carried
> cough medicine . . . and that kind of thing. [38]

"That kind of thing" was actually a great deal more than cough medicine.
According to lists of the contents, the nurses' midwifery bags "weighed
almost 42 pounds when packed"[39] and contained numerous items, as well
as a wide variety of drugs. Among the items contained in the bag were
"kidney basins, rubber sheets and aprons, newspapers, a cotton apron, cap
and gown, sterile gloves, Lysol, alcohol, hypodermic syringe, catheters,
clamps and scissors"—everything needed for a delivery.

Drugs included in the saddlebag pack were "morphine, codeine, quinine, cascara, aspirin, chloral hydrate, brandy, castor oil, magnesium sul-
phate, silver nitrate, ergotrate, caffeine, and sodium benzoate"—all medicines that the FNS nurses were authorized to give according to the
*Routines.* The nurses could give other medicines "at their discretion for
discomfort and vague pains of all sorts."[40] These medicines included
aspirin, ichthyol, bismuth, castor oil, sulphur, unguentine, Vaseline,
senna, milk of magnesia, ipecac, rhubarb and soda, boric acid, zinc, and a
few others.[41]

## Furnishing Drugs

Much like the nurses at Henry Street, the FNS nurses dispensed and
administered these over-the-counter remedies (widely used by middle-
class women in their homes) to the poor families in Appalachia, some of

whom no doubt had never even heard of the medicines. In other cases, they gave proprietary medicines like morphine and codeine according to standing orders.[42] The nurses were entrusted to carry these highly addictive, controlled drugs, limited to physicians' and dentists' use by the 1914 Harrison Narcotic Act, only out of necessity to provide pain relief to a patient, or to treat a patient for shock caused by pain, "when a doctor could not be had." Because Part II of the 1917 *Frank v. South* Kentucky ruling stated that nurses could give drugs "in the absence of the physician but in accordance with his directions," the FNS nurses had the legal back-up they needed to do so.[43]

The guidelines for the use of narcotics were specific and required the nurse to carefully document their use and report the usage to the physician. For example, the 1928 edition of *Routines* stated that morphine sulfate should be given for shock, with doses ranging from "$1/_8$ to $1/_4$ grains, depending on the weight of the patient." It also recommended that for "acute chest conditions, codeine $1/_4$ to $1/_2$ grain doses should be administered for pain or great restlessness." The order followed with recommendations that if codeine was ineffective, the nurse should "give morphine in small doses."[44] In all instances, the nurse was expected to make an accurate assessment of the patient's condition before choosing to treat with an analgesic. Then, she was to use her own judgment to administer an appropriate dose.

Although the FNS nurses were not trained as nurse anesthetists, they carried "one can of ether"[45] in their saddlebags. They did *not* carry chloroform. Nonetheless, both drugs were discussed in the standing orders. Chloroform was only to be used in critical situations or in collaboration with a physician. (The doctor would bring the drug in his bag should he want to operate in the home.)  By contrast, the guidelines for using ether allowed the possibility that the nurse might give the drug on her own should a critical need arise. The *1928 Routines* were clear in this regard, warning the nurse against the use of chloform, but recognizing the fact that she might have to give it in an extreme emergency:

> Warning! If a nurse is asked by a doctor to give an anesthetic, she is to go ahead and he, of course, assumes responsibility. The occasion will very rarely arise when she will be called upon to give chloroform in the absence of a doctor. Nothing short of an extreme necessity justifies her in giving even a few whiffs, because of the great danger of chloroform to the heart. Ether is a safer drug. Great care should be taken with open fires and lamps where ether is used.[46]

The FNS nurses also used herbal remedies—once again following standing orders. For example, the 1928 *Routines* recommended ginseng root, steeped into a tea, for the treatment of infant colic, and black cohosh, or "rattleweed," for the alleviation of menstrual cramps. The *Routines* also contained recipes for homemade cough syrups. The 1936 edition authorized the FNS nurses to mix the medication as needed (essentially serving as pharmacists), directing them to:

> Put three tablespoons of dried or fresh horehound leaves and stalks in 1½ pints of water. Boil about ½ hour and strain. Add ½ pint honey. If unable to get honey, use brown sugar, ½ lb and boil ½ hour. Add ipecac in the proportion of 2 teaspoons to 1 ounce of the above mixture. Give 1 teaspoon every three hours for an adult patient. . . . [47]

The routine outlined by the medical committee for the treatment of boils and abscesses not only reflected the physician's attempts to place some limits on the nurses' practice (she was not to perform any treatment remotely similar to surgery), but also reflected their sensitivity to the widespread use of home remedies in the "Hoot Owl Hollers":

> The nurse not infrequently has to handle these [boils and abscesses] when it is not possible to get a doctor. . . . It is better for her to avoid opening [them] with a knife if this is possible. She may use such local treatments as ichthyol, antiphologistin, home-made poultices of corn meal etc and fomentations."[48]

Clearly the Medical Advisory Committee preferred that the FNS nurses avoid what they considered to be surgical procedures, in this case, piercing the boil or abscess. Perhaps they had had some bad experiences in the field and were aware of the complications that could ensue should the nurse attempt to lance a boil. Perhaps they were simply defending their territory. Either way, the physicians clearly preferred that the nurse use the home remedies.

Thus, using the *Routines* to ensure that they worked "in accordance with the physician's directions," the Frontier nurses not only provided midwifery services but also treated everything from snake bites, gunshot wounds, sore throats, and earaches, to acute abdominal pain, diphtheria, and typhoid fever.[49] In addition, they sutured lacerations; applied salve to boils, shingles, and burns; and treated elderly patients for such conditions as pneumonia, chest pain, and congestive heart failure.

## Diagnosing

The physicians who supervised the FNS nurses expected them to make clinical diagnostic decisions and treat the patients accordingly. It did not make sense to have a manual of standing orders if the nurses couldn't determine what illness the patient had and therefore which orders to follow. Typically physicians made a "working diagnosis"—determining the condition that was suspected to be the most likely cause of the patient's symptoms. Working alone in the remote Appalachian Mountains, the nurse had to use the same decision-making process the physicians used. It didn't matter to the physician advisory committee that the nurses were technically practicing medicine. The physicians were still in control, because the nurses reported to them and followed guidelines the doctors had written. Besides, the difficulties of travel and communication made it impossible for the physicians to reach patients in the isolated, backwoods area.

Whether or not the nurses called the decision-making process diagnosing, they were, in fact, making clinical assessments of the signs and symptoms they saw and acting on them. Writing to her colleague and friend Dr. Josephine Hunt, Mary Breckenridge questioned her own ability to diagnose—despite all evidence that she had already ruled out three possible diagnoses and was doing as well as the doctor she summoned in determining a fourth. Even more importantly, Breckenridge knew the limits of her abilities and when to seek further consultation.

> We have another woman, [with a] seven month old baby, very aenemic [sic], feet badly swollen, rapid pulse (122 sitting down any old time)—cannot get a diagnosis on her. Urine tested four times, no albumin. Stools sent off, no hookworms. Hazard doctor . . . examined heart and lungs and found nothing to account for her condition, but ordered digitalis to slow down the heart. Could we send her down . . . ? She can leave the baby who is flourishing. . . . [50]

In this case, Breckenridge had already made three possible diagnoses: (1) that the patient may have had an anemia; (2) that she may have had kidney failure as would have been evidenced by albumin in her urine; and (3) that she may have had hookworms. Acting on these differential diagnoses, Breckenridge had already sent off urine and stool for laboratory tests and received negative reports. She had subsequently ruled out two of her initial diagnoses—kidney failure and hookworms. Now, she was left with a patient, seven months postpartum, who had signs and symptoms of heart failure (probably postpartum cardiomyopathy). She knew that a heart rate of 122 "any old time" was not good. She also knew that she could not identify the underlying diagnosis, and called in a physician. The local physician may or may not have been able to diagnose the condition, either, but he did prescribe an appropriate drug—digitalis—to slow and strengthen the heart. Breckenridge, aware that the woman needed a complete diagnostic work-up, was referring the patient to the doctors in Lexington. Her care was safe, appropriate, and competent.

Not every case was quite so dramatic. Much of what the FNS nurses handled were minor illnesses like colds and sore throats. However, in these remote mountain hollows, even a sore throat could prove lethal—especially if it turned out to be diphtheria. Accordingly, the physicians gave the FNS nurses explicit directions to treat for diptheria if they even suspected that diagnosis. In the *Routines,* the physicians outlined the signs and symptoms to help the nurses make the diagnosis in their absence. The 1928 *Medical Routines* reflected the physicians' awareness of both the high incidence of mortality in untreated cases of diphtheria and the reality of backwoods medical practice:

> When there are membranes [in the patient's throat], of course suspect diptheria and when in doubt use anti-toxin. A doctor must be had if it is humanly possible, but unless he can be had almost at once, do not wait before giving not less than 10,000 units [of anti-toxin], and if the case is advanced, give 20,000 units. Diphtheria moves with such rapidity that it is better to chance giving anti-toxin to a child with tonsillitis that to wait for a diagnosis if conditions are very suggestive. . . . [51]

Providing immediate access to treatment could save lives in this remote area of the country. Recognizing this reality, the local physicians were willing to allow nurses to expand their scope of practice to include diagnosis and treatment.

## Preventive Medicine or Nursing?—Overlapping Practice Areas

Less typical of the standing orders were those ordered by the medical committee for the care of an infant with diaper rash. To treat "sore buttocks or skin," the doctors prescribed the use of "bismuth and castor oil or zinc ointment . . . with ichthyol ointment . . . as an alternative."[52] Prescribing these drugs was well within the scope of medical practice. However, the physicians also ordered the nurse to "teach the family how to wash diapers." The task of teaching hygienic practices (e.g., washing diapers and sheets, ventilating the room, etc.) had long been considered within the purview of nursing.[53] In writing these orders, the doctors were prescribing preventive medicine; they were also "practicing" nursing. In this situation, the scope of medical and nursing practice overlapped.[54]

Another instance in which the physician's work overlapped with the nurse's responsibilities was in the orders they gave for "Care of the Baby at Delivery." Most of these orders were reasonably within the boundaries of the medical profession, including orders to clamp and cut the cord, and to place silver nitrate in the infant's eyes. However, other orders overlapped with nursing, and the experienced nurse-midwives knew what they should do without having physicians tell them. Certified nurse-midwives did not need medical orders telling them to "oil the baby but do not wash until next visit . . . weigh . . . dress . . . and put to the breast for five minutes."[55] Nor did they need orders to "give the mother at least one complete bath during the first ten days . . . and put her bed in order each day."[56] The nurses were well acquainted with these nursing activities. They had been taught the basics of nursing care in their training programs. They had also been taught specifics about care of the mother and the newborn in their postgraduate midwifery courses. On the one hand, the doctors were being too prescriptive, describing every detail of the care they wanted implemented in the maternity cases. On the other hand, they could not be blamed for their overly solicitous instructions. They had seen the complications and the deaths that had resulted when untrained granny midwives had delivered the mountaineers' babies. Besides, the physicians may have been unfamiliar with the nurses' knowledge base and expertise and had yet to trust them. Moreover, the doctors were also trying desperately to decrease maternal and infant deaths.

## Working with the Community

According to FNS assistant director Mary Willeford, the Frontier nurses worked "through" the community and not "for" it. Each nursing center had a local committee composed of "leading citizens in the district." The nurses met with the members twice a year, reporting on their work and discussing various problems.[57]

In addition to working with the local committee, the nurses approached each family individually, always aware that they were guests in the highlanders' homes. The nurse was particularly careful to establish rapport with the mother. Recounting her experiences in an article in the *American Journal of Nursing,* nurse-midwife Vanda Summers was careful to describe this process, writing:

After a quarter of an hours' ride, we come to our next home. The baby
is just six months old. We sit talking for a while in front of the fire,
inquiring after the baby's health and habits, et cetera, and then we discuss with the mother the importance of giving the baby its diphtheria
"shot," and ask her to bring it up to us on a clinic day. . . . The mother may want to get permission from the father, the grandfather, the
grandmothers, the uncles, the aunts, or even the cousins beforehand.[58]

Part of establishing rapport with the mountain families was the nurses'
willingness to use herbal and other home remedies with which the highlanders were already familiar. After identifying the herbs and acquiring
knowledge about their uses, the FNS nurses used them to alleviate symptoms of conditions such as poison ivy, toothaches, and colds. They also
used various remedies to reduce inflammation, relieve constipation, and
treat diarrhea and numerous other conditions.

Commonly used wild herbs included ginseng, sassafras, poke root,
Indian Arrowwood, cohosh, pleurisy root, nettles, and wild ginger.[59]
The FNS nurses frequently used ginseng root, steeped into a tea, to
treat babies for colic and girls for menstrual cramps. In the *FNS
Quarterly Bulletin,* Mary Breckenridge noted several other herbal
remedies nurses employed, including black cohosh, or "rattleweed,"
to both alleviate pain and regulate flow in young girls' menstrual periods, and "to strengthen the muscles that help in child birth" for pregnant women. In the latter case, the "whole root was boiled in water
for twenty minutes, and the water was then drained off. About half a
tea cup full was drunk twice a day."[60]

Upper respiratory conditions were particularly responsive to homemade remedies. According to Breckenridge, another commonly used herb
was nettles. "The root, steeped into a strong tea is drunk by the cupful several times a day. It is used for 'spring nettles' or hives, whelps, and knots."[61]
The FNS nurses frequently used pleurisy root (commonly known as milk-
weed or butterfly weed), steeped into a tea, to treat "side pleurisy." For
coughs, they administered the bark of Indian arrowwood, skinned off,
boiled, and made into cough syrup with honey.[62]

Grindelia and potash were used to treat poison ivy. According to the
1928 *Routines,* the nurse was directed to: "paint parts with fluid extract
of grindelia or scrub area open with soap and water, using sterile brush
and apply permanganate of potash strength 1–1,000. . . ."[63] The plant
"Deadly Night Shade" could also be used as a remedy for poison ivy.
Preparation of the herb was the first step in the treatment process.
Directions included: "Beat up the leaves with sweet milk until the mix-
ture is 'right green' and apply externally for poison ivy. Wash the bad

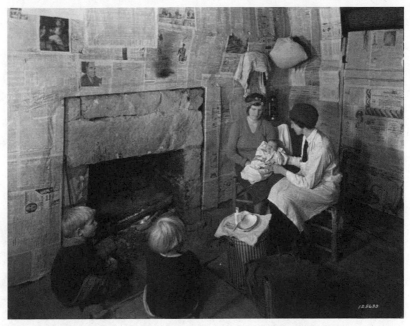

Figure 3.4: Nurse teaching well-baby care. Caufield & Shook Collection, Ekstrom Library, University of Louisville

places and then wrap them up. Never use internally because Deadly Night Shade is a poison."[64]

Diarrhea, called "running-off, or flux or bloody flux," was especially prevalent among babies and young children in the poverty-stricken Appalachian region. To treat it, the nurses administered a tea of "Blue John," made from a little vine found around barns,[65] or "Goose Grass," another little vine which could be "boiled until strong, then cooled and drunk three times a day."[66]

The FNS nurses applied poke root, an anti-inflammatory, to treat "any kind of pain," but particularly "rheumatism." The root was roasted, split open, and bound to the site. An alternative was to administer a drink of poke berries mixed with whiskey.[67]

In addition to herbs, the Kentucky nurses frequently employed common household spices as medications. For example, cloves, used as a spice in cooking, were used to treat toothache. Note the following guidelines for treatment in the 1930 FNS *Medical Routine*: "if both heat and cold cause pain, the condition is an acute pulpitis and oil of cloves should be dropped into the cavity."[68] Clearly both physicians and nurses were not adverse to using whatever was available and whatever worked.

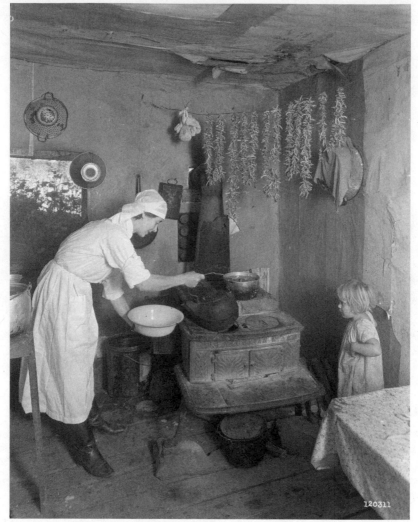

Figure 3.5: FNS nurse at stove. Caufield & Shook Collection, Ekstrom Library, University of Louisville

## The Economic Depression

The grim realities of the Great Depression increased the need for services in Leslie County in the 1930s. The already impoverished residents were particularly devastated when a year-long, severe drought ruined local crops and the timber industry—their two main income sources. Indeed, rural communities often fared worse than towns and cities during the period of the Depression. Lack of money to pay for medical services forced many people to go without them, and the highlanders were no exception.[69]

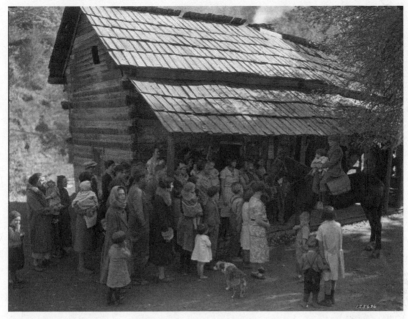

Figure 3.6: Highlanders at FNS clinic. Caufield & Shook Collection, Ekstrom Library, University of Louisville

Breckenridge's nurses responded—providing food, shoes, and clothing in addition to nursing services.[70] According to a draft of an article written for the *New York Times,* May 13, 1931, the nurses continued to make visits in the "holler" despite their dwindling sources of funding:

> They [the nurses] could not refuse help to any. Last winter they found families destitute—the chickens, pigs and cow long since sacrificed, the children barefoot in the snow. They drew on their dwindling funds for four quarts of milk a week for each child and 700 pairs of shoes and charged it up to "preventive work." . . . [71]

Despite the economic difficulties, the FNS nurses still held clinics to provide health services, and they still visited patients in their homes. And their outreach grew. By May 1934, the FNS nurses had made 161,832 home visits and seen 115,601 in the clinics.[72]

Since the inception of the FNS, the nurses had delivered over 2,000 infants with only 48 stillbirths and no maternal deaths owing directly to obstetrical causes. In the first 1,000 cases, the FNS nurses had two maternal deaths, both caused by chronic heart disease. In the second thousand deliveries, they had no maternal deaths "from any cause whatsoever."[73] In addition to maternity cases, the FNS nurses gave "over 68,000 inoculations and vaccination for such diseases as typhoid, diphtheria, influenza, pneumonia, smallpox, and tetanus. Three-thousand and fifty-four sick cases (not including midwifery) were cared for in their homes and all except 166 recovered."[74] At the close of the ninth fiscal year, the FNS was caring for 1,146 families, including 256 babies, 1,139 preschool children, 2,243 school-aged children, and 2,337 adults.[75] Clearly the FNS nurses were providing care to thousands of patients in the impoverished community. Without a doubt, part of what they did lay within the domain of public health nursing, like giving inoculations and doing health teaching. The remainder was a combination of standard home care, primary medical care, and midwifery services.

By 1936, the FNS had a new medical director, John H. Kooser, MD, a physician who was supportive of the nurses expanding their skills and their scope of practice.[76] In fact, Kooser taught the nurses how to identify various physical findings to aid in their clinical assessments, and he occasionally requested that they administer ether during complicated deliveries.[77]

In contrast to Kooser's liberal approach and willingness to have the FNS nurses expand their role, the physicians who wrote the *Medical Routines* became gradually more conservative as the years progressed. Careful to acknowledge—albeit indirectly—that the FNS nurses were working in an expanded role, the foreword of the 1936 edition of *Medical Routines* reiterated the hardship under which the FNS nurses worked and authorized routines so that the nurses could "meet medical emergencies and carry on adequately until a physician can be obtained."[78] In other words, if obtaining a physician's services was impossible, nurses could do whatever they needed to do to care for the patient. Indeed, "carrying on adequately" often meant dispensing and furnishing drugs, including narcotics as well as other medicines.

In their 1936 *Routines*, the FNS advisory committee made it explicitly clear that narcotics were to be controlled, writing: "As a general rule, narcotics must not be given unless ordered by a physician. However, occasions do arise for exceptions and these are given below."[79] What followed was a list of conditions in which "one dose of morphine" could be administered when a physician was not available. These included: gastric or pulmonary hemorrhage, "severe gunshot cases," childbirth, acute abdominal pain, and shock. And in all cases, the 1936 guidelines mandated that the nurse "be in attendance for at least four hours following the administration of the narcotic." In addition, she was required to "report in writing to the medical director her administration of narcotics for such cases."[80]

## Collaboration and Professional Boundary Issues

Despite the conservative trend, the FNS advisory committee continued to approve and publish new editions of their standing orders, and the FNS nurses continued to use them. The advisory committee even expanded the number of drugs the nurses could give, adding new medications to the protocols each year. By the 1940s, after the sulfonamides and penicillin were widely accepted in practice, the *Medical Routine* authorized the FNS nurses to give these antibiotics.[81] The Frontier nurses had a great deal of autonomy in implementing the standing orders. In addition to specified doses of penicillin or tetracycline, the nurse could also "give symptomatic treatment, i.e.: Pyralgin for fever, aspirin for pain, phenergan for vomiting, etc. as needed."[82] In this case "etc." could cover most anything else in the *Routines*.

In 1948, Mary Breckenridge and Alexander J. Alexander, MD (formerly chairman of the 1925 Kentucky Committee for Mothers and Babies), collaborated in writing the standing orders, as is evidenced in Alexander's letters regarding the dosage of Trisulfin. In one letter dated 10 July, 1948, Dr. Alexander responded to Breckenridge's request that he specify doses on a child's *age* rather than on the child's *weight* because the FNS nurses had no scales on which to weigh patients. After writing the new orders, Alexander added, "If this [procedure] is not entirely satisfactory, I would suggest that you blue pencil [edit] this letter . . . [and return it to me]."[83] As reflected in the letter, the sense of trust established between these two professionals, working together to provide care to the poverty-stricken highlanders, is palpable.

Despite the growing sense of trust and collegiality between the FNS nurses and the local physicians, by the mid-twentieth century the physician advisory committee was increasingly concerned over professional boundary issues. In fact, the wording of the instructions to the nurses in the *Medical Routines* becomes increasingly precise with each edition. For example, the introduction to the 1948 version explicitly states that FNS nurses were to work *only* within the guidelines provided. According to that edition:

> The routines set forth in this book are the orders given by the physicians of the Medical Advisory Committee of the FNS for the use of nurses in the service. They must be followed exactly. No other medications or treatments may be used. . . . In a grave emergency you may act according to your own judgment, but must report the case in full to the Medical Director.[84]

The orders also became increasingly complicated. "Standing Orders" for children with "follicular tonsillitis, severe type" included:

> Under 5 years:
> 300,000 units Procaine Penicillin IM stat, then start 125 mgm oral penicillin for ten days (Pentide, Pen-Vee K, Compocillin, TID).
>
> 5–10 years:
> 600,000 units Procaine Penicillin stat, then start oral penicillin as above.
>
> Over 10 years:
> 600,000 units Procaine Penicillin stat, start 250 mg oral Penicillin TID x 10. If the patient has a sensitivity reaction to Penicillin, give Tetracycline as below . . . if a child is not tolerating Tetracycline, substitute Erythromycin . . . or Pediatric drops of Achromycin. . . . When acute otitis media is also present . . . be sure to give ear drops.[85]

To interpret these orders, the nurse would have to be familiar with the types of penicillin and how they were given, the signs and symptoms of penicillin reaction, and the signs and symptoms of otitis media (a middle ear infection) in addition to the usual understanding of abbreviations such as "stat" (the Latin for "statim," or immediately), "IM" for intramuscular, "TID" for three times a day, and other abbreviations.

Changes in leadership in the advisory board, an increase in medical knowledge, the rapid development of new drugs, and the changing economic climate from the depression to the war years all played a part in accounting for the stricter controls on the FNS nurses' practice over time. Whatever the case, by mid-century the FNS medical advisory board was attempting to reinforce traditional boundaries on the nurses' scope of practice. Nonetheless, the FNS nurse-midwives would not be deterred from their practice and their educational mission to prepare other nurse-midwives. As Assistant Director Mary Willeford noted in her annual report for 1934:

> In regard to our plans for the future we have two specific aims. The first is to complete our originally planned demonstration area. . . . Our second is to use our territory as a training field for the preparation of nurses as midwives for other isolated sections of the country. . . . There are other sections of America . . . where graduate nurses trained as midwives are needed in maternal and infant care.[86]

By 1939 that goal would become a reality, when the Frontier Nursing Service opened what one FNS nurse, Dorothy Buck, called its "training course in midwifery and frontier technic for graduate registered nurses," in response to the loss of many of the British nurse-midwives who returned to England because of the war.[87]

By the next year, as a result of their efforts in education and in advertising, there were twenty-two nurses on staff at the Frontier Nursing Service. Moreover, Breckenridge met her goal to have the FNS showcased. In fact, visitors came from all over the world, including "Mexico, China, South Africa, Afghanistan, and Scandinavia," to see the "pioneer demonstration service of 'what can be done to give a country of poor people and difficult travel an inclusive nursing program.'"[88] Meanwhile, concurrent with the FNS nurses' work in the eastern United States providing access to care for poverty-stricken, rural white descendants of European immigrants, the Bureau of Indian Affairs field nurses were providing much the same medical and nursing services to the Navajo Indians in the West—a population that was not considered to be the "worthy poor."

# Chapter 4

# "My Treatment Was Castor Oil and Aspirin"

## Field Nursing among the Navajo People in the Four Corners Region, 1925–1955

December 3, 1931

Dear Emily,

. . . Lest you think I simply gossip with the neighbors, I will tell you of a typical day's work in my dispensary.

Man—(trachoma) eyes treated.

Baby—with diarrhea, diet and treatment outlined to mother.

Ute woman—aspirin for headache, cathartic—too much Yeibicai [traditional winter night ceremonial chant around a huge pinon fire].

Woman—ear irrigated to remove louse. Abdominal tumor discovered.

Man—complaining of pain in chest. Suspected nothing serious. Found he really wanted to sell me some mutton!

Child—extensive impetigo on face. Allowed the removal of scabs and the application of ointment without a murmur.

[Indian name]'s baby to hospital: Pneumonia—died later.

Hogan visited—Old man [name]—Chill last night, pain in chest, general aching, headache, temperature 101. Refuses to be taken to hospital. Visited Hogan the next day. [name of Indian] not at home—out herding sheep in the rain! Rumor later reported his complete recovery.

Man—ammoniated mercury ointment for three children with impetigo.

Woman—badly abscessed gums. Local treatment. To go to hospital for treatment.

Man—"toothache medicine": (oil of cloves) for wife.

Child—treated for impetigo.

[name of Indian] mother—cough syrup.

[name of Indian] wife—liniment.[1]

Elizabeth Forster

Like other field nurses working for the Bureau of Indian Affairs (BIA) in the first half of the twentieth century, public health nurse Elizabeth Forster had initially hoped to avoid giving medications. She wanted to distinguish the nurse's role—that of health promoter and case finder—from that of BIA physicians, who in the past had been known for dispensing pills.[2] Public health nurses were supposed to do health teaching and *assist* the physicians. Instead, Forster found herself alone, making diagnoses and treating patients. Writing on December 3, 1931 to her friend Emily, Elizabeth Forster gave the brief account above of a day's work in her dispensary. She gave little explanation, writing matter-of-factly about the care she provided. It was becoming routine for her to diagnose and treat commonly occurring conditions like trachoma, ear infections, and impetigo.

Forster, an experienced public health nurse, was working as a field nurse among the Navajo Indians in Red Rock, Arizona. Red Rock, a trading post, was located in a remote area of the Navajo reservation in the Four Corners region of the United States, where Colorado, New Mexico, Utah, and Arizona meet.

The best thing about Red Rock was that it had an abandoned mission hospital that could serve as Forster's home and clinic for her eighteen-month stay.[3] The old adobe brick hospital, previously owned by the Presbyterian church, was now government property, and the New Mexico Association of Indian Affairs superintendent, E. R. McCray, had promised that the building would be made ready for Elizabeth Forster's arrival. However, when she arrived in early November of 1931, Forster found that nothing had been done.[4] Instead, she had to live in two tiny rooms heated only by a small stove. For the entire month of November, Foster waited for the government to deliver fuel and renovate the mission to create a clinic room. With the exception of the delivery of a small bed and dresser mid-month, nothing was done, and Forster had to treat patients in her tiny kitchen.[5] Finally, in early December, the Indian Affairs agency delivered a supply of wood and coal, just in time for the cold winter ahead. Carpenters also renovated the mission to create a small dispensary. That month alone, Forster treated 138 Navajo patients.[6]

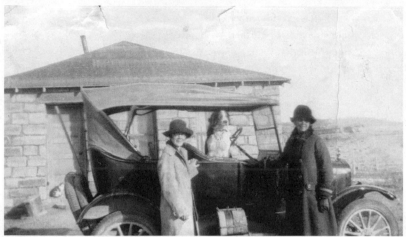

Figure 4.1: Elizabeth Foster with Model-T Ford, 1925. NAU-CL, BBWC

## The Federal Initiative

Forster's work at Red Rock was part of an experimental public health program sponsored by the New Mexico Association of Indian Affairs. It was
also part of a major federal government initiative to provide health care to
American Indians on reservations throughout the United States. The initiative began in 1849 with the transfer of the Bureau of Indian Affairs
from the War Department to the Department of the Interior, an act
designed to emphasize the nonmilitary aspects of Indian administration,
one of which was the provision of civilian medical services on the reservations. Within twenty-five years, about half of the Indian reservations had
a doctor, and by 1900, there were eighty-three physicians employed on
reservations.[7] However, the number was hardly sufficient. At no time during the late nineteenth and early twentieth century were there enough
doctors to meet the Indians' needs. In fact, the available Bureau doctors,
some of whom had little medical training, had such heavy case-loads that
they could do little more than issue pills. Adding to that problem, there
were no nurses. According to an early descriptive account of its history, the
BIA did not employ nurses until the 1890s, when they hired a few to work
in the Indian boarding schools.[8]

By 1900, the BIA had built several hospitals and had increased the
number of boarding schools on the reservations. In 1911, Congress appropriated $40,000 for general health services to Indians, the first significant
appropriation of its kind.[9] Then, in 1913, Congress ordered a public
health survey to identify the Indians' health care problems. According to

their findings, the most pressing need was for better sanitation. The report also called for more hospitals, better qualified and better paid physicians, and the employment of field nurses (RNs with public health training) to provide care for patients outside the hospitals. The major emphasis, however, according to a 1913 USPHS report, was on preventing contagious diseases that could spread to white Americans.[10] Based on these findings, Congress appropriated $90,000 to the Bureau of Indian Affairs, mostly for the control of trachoma and tuberculosis, the Indians' two most significant health problems.[11]

Despite the report's recommendations, prior to 1925 the BIA continued to hire minimally qualified field matrons rather than public health nurses to care for patients in the community. These untrained field matrons, working against overwhelming odds for minimal pay, were supposed to teach better sanitation and hygiene, provide emergency nursing services, and give medicines for minor illnesses.[12] However, owing to their lack of health care training and minimal qualifications, the matrons' work was often of inconsistent and often poor quality. According to a later report:

> No schooling [for field matrons] was required until 1924 when applicants were required to have the equivalent of an eighth grade education. . . . In 1916, applicants were required only to answer fully what experience, if any, they had in (a) cookery, (b) household sanitation, (c) sewing, (d) care of the sick, (e) care and feeding of infants, (f) home gardening . . . (g) social work and reform, slum, civic betterment or similar work.[13]

The skills needed for their work far exceeded the field matrons' capabilities. In fact, as a report on the Indian administration noted: "the types of service outlined for them would tax the most modern public health nurse, social case worker, and farm demonstration agent combined. . . ."[14] Nonetheless, it would take several more major studies followed by Congressional appropriations of funds before the Bureau employed licensed registered nurses were employed.

The continuing problems of the Bureau of Indian Affairs were finally on a Congressional agenda in the early 1920s. In 1921, Congress passed the Snyder Act, authorizing federal funds for health services to Native American tribes.[15] The funds were part of the peace treaty agreement made between the Indians and the US government as part of the government's compensation for its treatment of the Indians in the nineteenth century. Instead of using the funds to set up field clinics, the BIA built more hospitals. The problem was that the Navajos did not use hospitals, as they believed death lay within the hospital walls, and therefore the buildings were filled with evil spirits, *"Ch'iindis."*[16]

In an attempt to better meet the Indians' needs, in 1922 the Office of Indian Affairs commissioned the American Red Cross to conduct a survey of the health needs on the reservations, and in 1924, two years after they began the study, the Red Cross recommended "the immediate establishment of an organized public health nursing service as part of the Indian health program."[17] As a result, three trained Red Cross nurses were assigned to be visiting nurses on the Navajo reservation in a trial program. The experiment was a success, but it would take years to get the nursing service up and running because of a lack of money.[18] According to a 1928 report four years after the initial Red Cross recommendations, the "organization of nursing work in the Indian service" had not been "thoroughly established as yet."[19] In fact, numerous positions remained unfilled. That year, according to the same report, there were "25 public health nurse positions, 13 traveling surgical nurse positions and 115 hospital and sanatorium (TB) positions" available.[20]

## *The Meriam Report* and the Field Nurses

About the same time—in the mid-1920s—US Secretary of the Interior Hubert Work commissioned Lewis Meriam, a medical specialist employed by the Department of the Interior, to conduct a survey of the health services provided to the American Indians. Working with a prestigious staff of scientists and physicians from the Institute for Government Research, Meriam made a thorough investigation of the health services on the reservations and published the results in 1928 in a document entitled *The Problem of Indian Administration,* soon widely known as the *Meriam Report.* The report was graphic in its detail, describing extreme poverty, poor health and nutrition, and a lack of sanitation among the Indians. In addition, the Meriam report documented inadequate salaries for physicians and nurses, inadequate medical facilities, and minimal efforts toward preventive medicine. It also confirmed the fact that the two "great health problems" continued to be tuberculosis and trachoma.[21] According to the report, the Indian death rate from tuberculosis in Arizona was "15.1, more than seventeen times as high as the general rate for the country as a whole."[22] Of particular importance, the document "emphasized the need for stronger central supervision, more and higher-qualified field staff, and an accelerated public health program, including public health clinics on all reservations."[23] Part of that recommendation included a "plan to replace field matrons with public health nurses as rapidly as possible."[24]

Commissioner of Indian Affairs Charles J. Rhoads endorsed Meriam's findings. Under Rhoads's administration (1929–33), appropriations for education, health, and welfare increased. The increased funding was key to the implementation of a nursing service. Between 1924 and 1934, the number of field nurses employed by the government grew from three to ninety-eight. [25]

## Necessary Knowledge for Safe Care

Before nurses could be hired by the Bureau of Indian Affairs, they had to meet the civil service requirements for graduate nurse visiting duty. As of December 30, 1927, these requirements included:

> (1) completion of at least two years of a standard high school course, (2) graduation from a recognized school of nursing requiring a residence of at least two years in a hospital having a daily average of 50 bed patients or more . . . (3) not less than one year's institutional or two years private duty post-graduate experience in nursing, (4) evidence of state registration, (5) at least 4 months of post-graduate training in public health nursing or visiting nursing at a school of recognized standing . . . or [equivalent] experience. . . . [26]

In other words, the field nurses being hired had to have both public health educational preparation and postgraduate clinical experience. [27] The BIA administrators knew what the nurses would be asked to do, and they had to be assured that the nurses had the knowledge base they needed.

During this period of growth (1924–37), Elinor D. Gregg, RN, served as supervisor of nurses for the Indian Service. Her reports to the *American Journal of Nursing* document the fact that frequent transfers of nurses from one reservation to another were typical. The report also notes that some nurses chose to leave the service entirely. [28]

> *Transfers:* To Pyramid Lake San., Nevada, Louise J. Paddock; to Eastern Navajo Agency, New Mexico, Golden Blankenship; to Fort Hall Agency, Idaho, Katherine Gribneff; to Hopi Agency, Arizona, Naomi Tatum; to Tacoma Hospital, Washington, Josephine Heineman, and Julia Trabucco; to Southern Navajo Agency, Arizona, Mrs. Wauline H. Morse; to Sells Agency, Arizona, Mrs. Rosalie M. Vargas.
> *Separations*—three. [29]

Public health nurse Ida Bahl was the exception—she began to work for the BIA in 1934 and remained with the agency for twenty-three years. Bahl was well educated. She had a diploma from Mercy Hospital School of Nursing in Dubuque, Iowa, and a BSN in public health from the University of Washington School of Nursing. She also had clinical experience, which grew during her years in the Indian Health Service. Prior to her work in the Indian service, she had worked as an x-ray technician and as a private-duty nurse in Dubuque and Chicago. During the course of her employment with the BIA, Bahl worked in Arizona, Iowa, Oklahoma, California, Wisconsin, and New Mexico.[30] Later in her life, in the 1970s, she would survey the BIA nurses and physicians in order to document their work.

## The Field Nurse

Although the public health nurses who worked for the Bureau of Indian Affairs were generally more educated than the average nurse, in many ways they represented the majority of professional nurses of the era—they were women and they were single. Middle-class cultural norms identified nurses as women. The middle-class norms also defined women's primary role as wife and mother, creating the expectation that nurses would leave their jobs when they married or at least after they had their first child. The Bureau's policies also affected the choice of nurses who qualified for service. Single nurses were preferred. The severe shortage of separate housing on Indian reservations, resulting in the need to house nurses in dormitory residences, and the BIA regulation that "married women must present a statement of their home obligations," further ensured that the majority of BIA nurses would be single. However, as evidenced in the nursing supervisor's report, occasionally a married woman enlisted.[31]

The nurses who applied to the BIA were caucasian and middle class, not only because they represented the typical nurse of the era, but also because of the Bureau's discriminatory policies. The BIA was not open to African-American nurses. In addition, the agency required that the nurses supply their own uniforms ("navy blue or gray, washable"), and defray their own traveling expenses to the original post (significant for those traveling long distances west by train) and to alternate posts if the assignments were made at the nurse's request. These costs could be prohibitive for those who did not have adequate financial means.[32] Middle-class single white women were thus the norm in the BIA nursing service. Working among the Navajo people would be a completely new and challenging experience for these young women, as they were confronted with not only

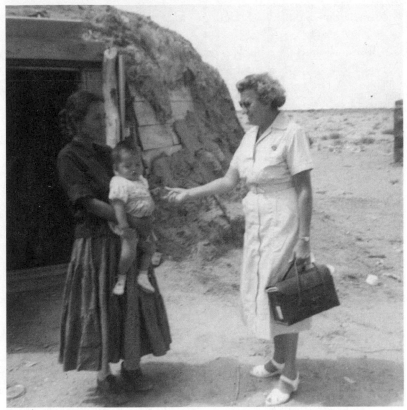

Figure 4.2: Navajo woman and child with Ida Bahl, 1961. NAU-BBWC, call # Nav. PH.92.14.2

poverty and isolation, but also with exotic customs, a peculiar language, and a strange culture.[33]

According to the field nurses' diaries and letters, many of those who sought employment with the BIA were seeking adventure and travel.[34] Others, particularly in the early years of the Great Depression, were simply looking for salaried positions, as jobs for nurses in hospitals (as supervisors) and outside (as private-duty nurses) were scarce. Some were seeking freedom from the constraints of hospital nursing they had known as students, and they found it. Despite the agency's attempts to ensure that the nurses would continue to work under the supervision of chief nurses and physicians, and according to its bureaucratic policies, the realities of weather, geography, epidemics, and shortages of physicians demanded changes in the way care was delivered. Meanwhile, the freedom that the BIA nurses had as they practiced in remote areas of the country was unprecedented. According to Lewis

Meriam, although the nurses' training "was of a specialized character, sometimes considerably in advance of the physicians"[35] with whom they worked,
the BIA nurses faced legal and ethical dilemmas in the reality of their practice situation. As Lewis Meriam noted, "If she [the nurse] is to function at
all effectively, she must work more or less independently . . . in direct violation of all public health nursing ethics."[36]

## Difficult Conditions

One of the most isolated reservations to which nurses were assigned was
the Navajo reservation in the Four Corners region. There, the open desert,
inhabited by the nomadic, sheep-herding Navajo, was a world unlike any
other. The vast, empty lands, sparsely dotted with buttes and rocks, pin-
ion tress, and desert grasses, was home to more than 100,000 Navajos
returned there in 1868 after the failure of the "Long Walk" to Fort
Sumner, New Mexico in 1863.[37] Bounded by the Grand Canyon on the
west and extending east into New Mexico, the reservation encompassed a
harsh environment with little water. There, the Navajos lived in hogans
(one-room, octagonal, domed houses made of logs or mud), scattered over
great distances.

   One of the first complaints to surface in the field nurses' reports was
the difficulty of reaching the Navajo to provide care. Sometimes traveling
alone and sometimes accompanied by Indian drivers who also served as
interpreters, the nurses crossed the barren landscape from 800 to 2,500
miles per month in all types of weather.[38] In the monsoon season that
began each year in July, sudden, unexpected torrential downpours could
cause flash floods over the "wash," wide, dry river beds capable of carrying raging torrents of water.[39] Sandstorms, high winds, and searing heat
further complicated travel.[40] Writing on August 1, 1932, Elizabeth Forster
described the difficulties that resulted when the field nurse in a neighbor-
ing district 90 miles away was on vacation and Forster had to cover for her:

> . . . when a rumor of a typhoid outbreak reached the hospital, I was
> asked to make as frequent visits as possible to the neighborhood to
> check on suspected cases. This I have done three times a week and
> in addition have been having a clinic at the Trading Post, 90 miles
> in another direction, once a week. . . . The sun blazes and no tree
> offers shade, the dust flies in smothering clouds, and yet we dread
> the coming of the seasonal rains which either cause us to stick in the
> mud or wait for hours on the bank of a wash while the water goes
> down. . . . [41]

Winter was no better, as blizzards could close roads indefinitely. In February 1932, Elizabeth Forster complained: "Life is proving strenuous just now with a Flu epidemic in progress and every effort to reach patients made difficult and prolonged by roads and weather. . . ."[42] Sometimes it was not the weather, but the sandy desert roads or the absence of roads that caused problems. According to field nurse Gladys Solverson's March 1936 report to the Bureau:

> This month we have had considerable illness on the reservation . . . 404 patients were visited and advised in their homes and 74 cases were seen at Trading Posts or Day Schools. We traveled 2025 miles and 110 hours over good and bad roads or more often, no road at all to reach these patients.[43]

When the roads were impassable, scheduled clinics could not be held.[44] Clinics could also be cancelled due to car trouble. Mary Eppich's terse entry in her March 1936 nursing report is typical: "On March 19, the car was out of commission and no clinic was made."[45] Twenty years later, the field nurses were still writing about their car troubles in their monthly reports to Washington, DC. Lillian Watson complained that the 1949 Ford sedan assigned to her was proving to be her biggest problem:

> It has been out of service four or five times during the month and now it is becoming routine . . . to take the car to the garage each morning before starting out to see what new trouble can be found. What a red letter day it would be if all the nurses were assigned new four wheel drive jeep station wagons![46]

The young female nurses had a right to complain—at least in part. The BIA officials assigned cars to male physicians, nonmedical agency superintendents, and other administrators before they allocated cars to nurses. The nurses received whichever were left. However, their situation was not all bad. Although the nurses did not get the best cars, they were assigned Indian drivers, as cultural norms required that the female nurses be accompanied when they traveled the reservation. In many instances, the fact that they had chauffeurs worked to the nurses' advantage. The Indian male chauffeurs not only drove the cars but also served as guides and interpreters. In doing so, they gave the nurses wide access to the Navajo people, introducing them to distant tribes. In addition, the drivers provided the nurses with companionship and additional pairs of hands. Sometimes they served as mechanics. According to one nurse:

When I think back over the times we were stuck in the mud, had engine trouble, flat tires, caught in flash floods driving mountain roads in the darkest night, I feel humble and grateful for having Mike as a helper.[47]

## Isolation and Autonomous Practice

When the Indian drivers were not available, the nurses made home visits unaccompanied. Because of the chronic physician shortage, the distances and the extreme weather conditions, doctors were frequently unavailable, and physician-nurse teams were not the norm. As a result, field nurses often found themselves alone making diagnoses and dispensing medicines.[48] Several nurses wondered or complained about being left on their own. Mary Zillitas mentioned that she was "desperately lonely in Shiprock."[49] Even Mary Eppich, who reported that she had been "brought to Red Rock in January of 1935 by Dr. Stephenson to work as a field nurse with him,"[50] lamented, "Have had several sick patients at the hogans and have wanted Dr. Stephenson to see them, but he has not made any clinics this month at Red Rock."[51]

Meanwhile, the Navajo people, who did not differentiate between doctors and nurses, expected to be treated with medicines. As Dorothy Loope noted: "I was forever trying to teach my people that I was a public health nurse, not a doctor—that I was there to help them learn how to prevent illness, not to treat it. But we often did treat it."[52]

## Diagnosing and Treating Illness

Because they were frequently on their own, the field nurses became adept at diagnosing and treating patients for a multitude of illnesses, whether it was legally and professionally acceptable or not. Three prevalent conditions they saw were tuberculosis (TB), trachoma, and infantile diarrhea. After seeing numerous cases of TB, the nurses became expert at making the diagnosis. In one instance, Mary Eppich identified the illness as soon as she saw the child, noting in her report: "Upon seeing the child, all symptoms of tuberculosis were evident."[53] The BIA nurses diagnosed and treated a myriad of other conditions, including colds, diaper rash, ear infections, pneumonia, venereal disease, burns, spider bites, diabetes, meningitis, appendicitis, breast abscesses, conjunctivitis, whooping cough, measles, chicken pox, impetigo, flu, acute poliomyelitis, and malnutrition.[54] Legally, their practice was covered by "standing orders" written

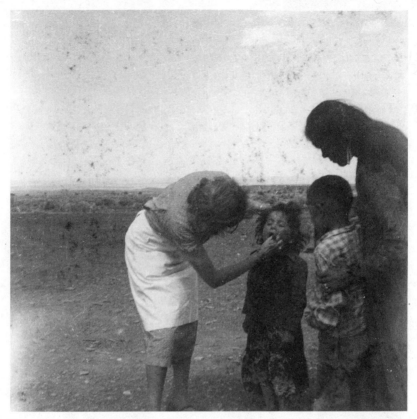

Figure 4.3: Ida Bahl examines Navajo girl, woman, and boy, 1955. NAU-CL, NAU.PH 92.14.5

ahead of time by the physicians with whom they worked. Like those developed for the Frontier Nursing Service and other public health nurses, these standing orders provided specific guidelines for the treatment of various problems the nurse might encounter. However, the guidelines were not all inclusive. Frequently the field nurses had to use their own expertise and clinical judgment. Demonstrating her trust in the nurses' ability to treat the patient appropriately, one physician made it clear that, after the fact, she would "write any order" the nurse needed."⁵⁵ That way, the nurse could feel secure that she would have the backup she needed to treat the patient as she saw fit.

Although they had the support of the BIA physicians, the field nurses' concerns about making medical diagnoses came through in their reports to the Bureau of Indian Affairs headquarters in Washington, DC. For example, in order to protect herself legally, Nena Seymour documented her diagnoses in her monthly report as "suspected whooping cough," and "suspected meningitis" rather than writing the more definitive diagnoses.[56] Diagnosing and treating patients independently was a new experience for the field nurses and clearly stretched their professional boundaries. According to Ruth Seawright, "There I was, 35 miles from the contract doctor and I had never given a patient 5 grains of aspirin without a doctor's orders."[57]

Despite their concerns about legal liability, the BIA nurses did whatever they had to do to care for the Navajo people. In April 1933, Elizabeth Forster saw 397 patients in her dispensary and made 65 hogan visits.[58] In May 1935, Nena Seymour made home visits to "76 different Hogans," and gave "the usual treatments" for sore throats, ear infections, cuts, impetigo and other commonly occurring diseases.[59]

In addition to visiting the hogans, the nurses conducted "nursing conferences," the initial intent of which was health education, not treatment. The purpose of these conferences was to instruct the Navajo women about infant and child care, sanitation, nutrition, and the importance of prenatal care. The conferences were also for the purpose of giving immunizations, making baby clothes, and conducting well-baby checkups.[60] However, in actuality, the conferences became "nurse-run" clinics, as the Navajo mothers would bring sick infants and children to the "conference" to be seen by the nurse. Reporting on her work at Teec Nos Pas in the Northern Navajo region in May 1931, Dorothy Williams described that reality. In fact, she referred to the conferences as "clinics":

> Five clinics held this week, three general and two baby clinics. Mothers bathed their babies and were given material to cut out and make gowns for baby. Preschool children were weighed, inspected and mothers advised [about] diets for underweights [sic]. . . . Fifty treatments given in dispensary.[61]

Once she had the facilities ready, Nena Seymour opened clinics in specific localities in order to decrease her own travel and that of the Navajos who migrated to the mountains for the summer. She also organized her day in order to care for the hundreds of Navajos who came to the clinic for treatment of trachoma, a highly contagious eye infection that was widespread on the reservation.

> My Mexican Springs dispensary is at last painted and I set up clinics. Routine trachoma treatments have been started. I have set aside 7:30–9:00 AM for trachoma treatments and other treatments each day . . . I have established a "Community Medical Center" up in the mountains for the summer.[62]

The Indians did not hesitate to ask the field nurses for eye medications, bypassing any attempt by the medicine men to treat this disease. Trachoma, aggravated by the hot, dry climate, dust, and wind of the desert, caused granular bumps on the inside of a patient's eyelids that caused excruciating pain when they scratched the cornea. Left untreated, the disease eventually resulted in blindness.

Apparently acknowledging that the white man's medicine relieved pain and itching, and helped them preserve their eyesight, the ever-practical Navajos willingly attended clinics, demanding treatment. The nurses, encountering numerous patients with the signs and symptoms of trachoma on a daily basis, quickly learned how to diagnose and treat the condition. Sometimes they confirmed the diagnosis with the physician before treating it. In March 1935, Mary Eppich reported that four trachoma patients were treated twice a week with "Silver Nitrate 2%" and were taught to drop "zinc solution 1% into their own eyes twice a day" on the days they did not come to clinic.[63] Covering herself legally in her report to Washington, Eppich also noted: "These were the orders of Dr. Johnson when I spoke to him on March 20, 1935."[64]

## The Nurses' Bag and "The Bag of Tricks"

The nurses carried their medicines with them, either in their black nursing bags or in what one of them called her "Box of Tricks," the box of medicines she carried with her in the car as she made home visits.[65] In these, the BIA nurses carried standard medical therapies used by physicians, druggists, and white, middle-class Americans in cities and towns throughout the United States. Like the medications used by the Henry Street Visiting Nurses and the Frontier Nurses in the 1920s and 1930s, these drugs provided symptomatic relief. Aspirin, castor oil, cough medicine, zinc oxide, eye drops, and Vaseline, all nonprescription drugs widely available in drugstores, were typical. For example, Mary Eppich reported using both castor oil and aspirin to treat a young child:

> [named child], 2 years old, a case of symptoms of Catarrhal fever with a temperature of 105, refused hospitalization was taken care of at the Hogan. Castor oil was given and aspirin Gr. 1 every four hours, plenty of water, no food for 24 hours. This child has a bad case of Otitis Media, which is carefully watched and treated in case a mastoid [sic] may result. Much improvement has been shown.[66]

In addition to castor oil, cod liver oil was also a favorite among BIA nurses and doctors in the Indian service during the 1920s and 1930s. The drug was particularly useful for malnourished children and patients with tuberculosis. As Mary Eppich recorded: "In the cases of tuberculosis where hospitalization has been refused, my only treatment is cod liver oil . . . and advice about rest, diet and especially taking care of other members of the family. . . ."[67] According to Lavinia Dock's 1921 *Materia Medica,* cod liver oil was "an alternative to the general nutrition in various disease conditions and is more truly a food than a medicine as it supplies the need of the tissues for fat."[68] No doubt, it improved the Navajo children's skin problems, because it supplied them with vitamins critically lacking in their diet, which often consisted only of "coffee and Navajo bread."[69] Because of the deficient nutrients, manly of the children suffered from impetigo, an itchy, contagious skin disease characterized by blisters that gradually formed a yellow-brown crust. Because the infection was also exacerbated by poor hygiene, Mary Eppich used a combination of treatments:

> Three severe cases of Impetigo were found in one Hogan. The treatment consists of washing with green soap, applying ammoniated mercury and bandaging. All three cases have shown much improvement. Also cod liver oil was given to them. . . .[70]

Another frequently used medication was silver nitrate. The nurses used the antiseptic solution to treat eye conditions such as conjunctivitis or as a prophylaxis in the eyes of a newborn. Argyrol was another commonly used eye medication. Mary Eppich recorded its use in children with measles:

> [two children's names] were found to have measles. Advised to keep warm, plenty of water and liquid diet, aspirin when necessary and castor oil. Argyrol 25% put into their eyes when I go to see them. . . .[71]

Eppich's treatment was symptomatic. It was all there was to offer. According to the 1903 edition of the *Physician's Handy Book of Materia Medica and Therapeutics,* the treatment of measles was to "follow general treatment for fevers, prescribing for symptoms as they arise."[72]

Despite the propensity to treat symptoms, not all of the drugs the field nurses dispensed were over-the-counter medications used for symptomatic relief. Ammoniated mercury ointment, mentioned by Mary Eppich as the treatment for impetigo and listed in Dock's 1921 *Materia Medica,* was a prescription drug commonly used for "treatment of skin diseases and irritations."[73] Elizabeth Forster also used it to treat impetigo. The BIA nurses also gave morphine and sleeping pills, which they carried with them for use in emergencies. In addition, after sulfanilamide and penicillin became available, the nurses used them to treat infectious illnesses. Sulfanilamide, in particular, was excellent for treating trachoma and revolutionized the care of this disease. By the 1940s, both nurses and physicians used penicillin to treat strep throat, chronic ear infections, venereal disease, pneumonia, and nephritis.[74]

## Working with the Contract Doctors

Although it may not have been often, the field nurses did work with physicians. On January 10, 1932, about eight weeks after her arrival in Red Rock, Forster wrote to her friend Laura Gilpin that she was collaborating with a physician on a weekly basis. (She also noted that she used food and shelter as a means of interesting the Navajos in attending the new clinic.)

> Have I told you that I am having clinics once a week with a doctor out from the hospital? The weather is so cold and my people have to come from such distances that I am preparing and serving soup for them, and my dispensary, warmed by a cheerful wood fire and advertising my soup in odoriferous fashion, is a popular place on clinic day. I strongly suspect many of them come for soup and not from need to see the doctor. I am, however, by means of this bait catching a good many cases which would not otherwise come to us for care: cases of trachoma, diseased tonsils, chronic appendicitis etc. . . . [75]

Forster was not the only nurse to work with a physician. According to one of Mary Eppich's reports, when Dr. Stephenson could make it to a clinic at Teec Nos Pas, he and Eppich treated fifty patients.[76] Eppich also worked with Dr. Elliot and, as evidenced in her report, clearly deferred to him when she did so:

> March 16–21: Four clinics held this week, large number of Navajos in for medicine and treatment. Dr. Elliott and myself [*sic*] attended the farmers meeting at Teec Nos Pas and he explained to the Navajos the reason for the children being vaccinated and having inoculation etc. and answered all the questions. . . .[77]

Other nurses worked with visiting physician specialists. Gladys Solverson, writing in April 1936, reported that she and Dr. Hancock had seen ninety-three patients in their trachoma clinic that month,[78] and Mollie Reebel wrote that "the clinics are being kept up regularly with Dr.

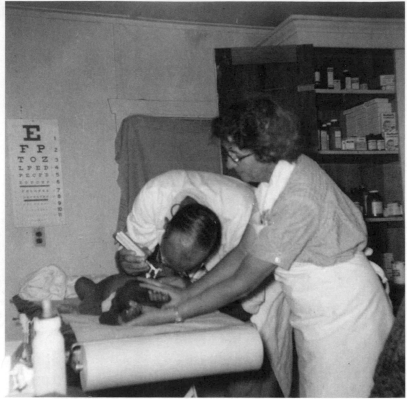

Figure 4.4: Ida Bahl and doctor examining child, 1955. NAU-CL, NAU.PH 92.14.3

Barklow in attendance."[79] Clearly, when the doctors were present, the nurses slipped into the much less autonomous (traditional) role of assistant.

Whether or not the nurses saw much of the physician with whom they were assigned depended on the circumstances in which they found themselves—including not only the geographic distance from the physician, the weather, the road conditions, and the availability of the physician, but also the doctor's willingness to work with nurses. Some, like Forster, Eppich, and Reebel, worked with doctors in cooperative arrangements. Another nurse had quite the opposite experience. According to Lydia King:

> . . . Our senior medical officer . . . is not in sympathy with field nurses and to quote him "looks forward to the day when there will be no field nurses in the Navajo Area,"—it all looks pretty discouraging from where I sit.[80]

Why this particular senior medical officer did not want nurses to work on the reservation is unclear. Evidence from the nurses' reports supports the fact that other doctors, working at the grassroots level, welcomed the nurses and trusted their judgment.[81] When conditions permitted, together they visited patients in their hogans, conducted specialty clinics and surgeries, and attended meetings on the reservations. Later, some praised the nurses' work as they reflected on the years of collaborative practice in the Indian service. Writing to Ida Bahl in the 1970s, BIA physician Charles S. McCammon was clear about his feelings on the subject: "There has never been any question that the public health nurse . . . was and still is the back bone of Indian community health programs. . . ."[82]

## Between the Contract Doctor and the Medicine Man

One of the most difficult tasks the nurses had to undertake in the BIA service was negotiating their role between the white American contract doctors and the Navajo medicine men. As historians Abel and Reifel have documented, the field nurses accepted without question the dominance of scientific American medicine.[83] Now, understanding the Navajo culture and the importance of balance and order to the Indians was essential in fostering a collaborative relationship and a sense of trust between the nurses and the people. Although not all nurses did so, many of the BIA nurses appreciated the fact that Navajo traditional healing ceremonies were at the foundation of their society and had to be incorporated into the care if any white man's treatment was to be accepted. According to Delores Young, who worked at a hospital in Crownpoint, New Mexico in 1945 and subsequently as a public health nurse in Tuba City, Arizona: "With the younger Indians who were undecided as to which medicine was the best, it was important to let them have both if they wanted it."[84] Another BIA nurse, Mary Zillatas, noted that she "tried to show the Indians that both cultures could be used to their advantage."[85] Both of these nurses worked according to recommendations written by Lewis Meriam: "The position taken . . . is that the work with and for the Indians must give consideration to the desires of the individual Indians."[86]

Therefore, rather than force "white man's medicine" on the Navajo, some field nurses tried to get the Indians to accept them as individuals first so that they then could introduce Anglo-American medicine, culture, health practices, and beliefs. The first step in this process was for the nurse to accept the Navajo culture. Many BIA nurses respected the Navajos' centuries-old customs and the medicine men's (Hataatii's) traditional practices, even though the nurses themselves did not always agree with the

Indians' beliefs. What the nurses could agree with was the Navajo' holistic perspective. The Navajos believed that "the system of life is one interconnected whole" and that "the whole human creature—body, mind and spirit," should be treated.[87] This holistic perspective was at the core of what nursing as a profession had been advocating since its inception. There were some significant differences, however, that were foreign to the increasingly scientific American nursing practice in the first half of the twentieth century. A major component of the Navajo medicine men's treatment involved "Sings," or "chantways," ceremonial chants that the Hataatii sang over the patient.[88] One of these, called "Beauty Way," was meant to restore balance to the patient. It was based on the Navajo belief that an imbalance or lack of harmony in any area of a person's life could cause illness.[89] Other ceremonial chantways included "Lifeway," "Blessingway," "Enemyway," "the Night Chant," "the Mountain Way," and "Shooting Way." Different chants were meant to cure different illnesses: a "Shooting Way" ceremony might be used to cure an illness thought to have been caused by a snake, lightning, or an arrow; a "Lifeway" was used to cure an illness caused by an accident; "Enemyway" healed an illness believed to be caused by the ghost of a non-Navajo.[90] An important part of one Sing, "the Night Chant" or "Yei-bi-chei," was an elaborate sand-painting created by the medicine man during the day of the ceremony. Some of the nurses attended these ceremonies and recorded their impressions, including the fact that sometimes (to their surprise) a cure took place! According to Ida Bahl:

> The medicine man spends days gathering materials and preparing them, and during this time a ceremonial Hogan is built by the family. The usual procedure is to clear the floor in the center . . . and cover it with clean white sand. . . . The medicine man or shaman . . . and his assistants . . . create figures of the Holy People, or the Yeis, and sacred plants in story designs. They use pulverized sandstone of various hues, charcoal, pollen, and meal, and let it slip through the fingers of the right hand . . . everything must be exactly right! . . . In the meantime, the patient prepares by taking a bath and shampooing the hair in yucca suds. Then the shaman gives an emetic. The patient sits beside a hot fire to induce profuse sweating . . . they muster the strength to go through the whole rite. . . . The patient is given a potion of herbs to drink and part of it is applied to the body. . . . Sand is transferred from each part of the painting to the same part of the patient's body . . . to absorb the might of the supernatural forces to avert evil and ill health. All the time, the shaman chants. . . . He finishes before sundown when the painting must be

erased. . . . Then they prepare for the ceremonial dances. . . . Often
a surprising and unexplained cure takes place.[91]

Some BIA nurses respected these beliefs and did not interfere with the
traditional care, even when they disagreed. According to Dorothy
Williams:

> Navajos requested me to visit a sick child in a hogan one day this
> week. When I got there I found that the child had a broken leg—
> compound fracture—and I advised hospital for child [*sic*] but the
> family said they had already sent for the medicine man and would
> send the child to hospital in a few days if he failed to cure the leg. I
> visited the hogan a few days later and found they were still having a
> "Sing."[92]

Although she may have been discouraged by the parents' refusal to send
the child to the hospital, Williams did not press the issue and instead waited for the medicine men to decide to do something different. Sometimes,
that delay was fatal. According to field nurse Lillian Watson, who worked
among the Navajo in the 1950s under the Indian Health Service:

> Attempts to persuade the mother of one two-year old boy, diagnosed
> as having military tuberculosis, to return him to the hospital failed
> and it was learned that the child died in the Hogan after receiving
> treatment by the grandfather who is reported to be a medicine
> man.[93]

## Collaborating with the Medicine Men

Not every medicine man denied white man's medicine (or in this case,
white women's therapies) to his patients. In fact, some accepted the nurses' therapy as adjunct treatments to the chants. According to Mary Eppich:

> [name], age 1 year, also has symptoms of Catarrhal Fever. A Sing is
> being held over him. My treatment was Castor Oil and Aspirin Gr. 1
> [grains 1] every four hours, plenty of water and not much food. . . . [94]

Clearly, some of the field nurses recognized the legitimate power of the
medicine men (Hataatii) within the community and the importance of
working with them rather than undermining their authority. Solveson
described the results of that collaboration, noting:

It has been gratifying to realize that we have gained the confidence of
several of the better known medicine men. We have been called frequently this month by the medicine men, both to their own homes
as well as to "sings," to consult regarding their patients. Frequently the
medicine man has advised the family to consider hospital care when
we recommended it. We have brought in a good number of patients
who had never seen the inside of a hospital before.[95]

The Hataatii's cooperation was essential to any consideration of hospitalization. And sometimes that cooperation was forthcoming. Robert
Trennert, who wrote extensively on government physicians' work with the
Navajo, noted that many of the medicine men believed that white man's
medicine was better in curing what they referred to as "white men's diseases"—for example, whooping cough, small pox, measles, tuberculosis.[96]
Because the Navajo community had invested the Hataatii with decision-
making power, the medicine men could decide to accept the white man's
ideas about treatment if their own treatment wasn't working. According to
Gladys Solveson:

Recently we advised an influential medicine man to hospitalize his
13 year old boy. The boy had been sick six days and had a temperature of 104 degrees. A "sing" was in progress and several medicine
men were present. After a discussion of about an hour and a half, the
medicine men decided to send the patient to the hospital. The father
accompanied his boy and watched his progress daily as he visited him
in the hospital. Recently, we sent him home well. It is to be hoped
his father has become better acquainted with hospital treatment and
that he has more confidence in our care of a patient.[97]

Although some BIA nurses shared information about illness with the
medicine men, attempting to educate them, their attempts were not
always successful. In one instance, Dorothy Williams tried to teach the
Hataatii the differences between chicken pox and impetigo. According to
her February 1936 report:

Several children came to school with chickenpox in Teec Nos Pas.
There is quite an epidemic. . . . The Navajos think it is impetigo and
come to the dispensary for ammoniated mercury to apply. . . . I tried
to explain to them the symptoms of chickenpox but they are quite
unable to understand contagious diseases.[98]

Over time, some of the nurses' effort paid off, particularly when they were accepting and nonjudgmental about cultural differences, which was not always the case, as has been well documented in Emily Abel's and Nancy Reifel's work.[99] In her final report to the National Association of Indian Affairs in 1933, Elizabeth Forster wrote:

> I believe that the Red Rock Navajos were beginning to accept me as a friend. . . . It was gratifying to have them voluntarily invite me to their ceremonies and sand paintings and to find the Medicine Men very willing to cooperate on increasingly frequent occasions.[100]

Working with people of a different culture and in harsh surroundings was not the only challenge the nurses and physicians faced. These professionals also had to question some of their own cultural norms, particularly the conviction—instilled in them early in their careers and reinforced by state medical practice acts—that only physicians could diagnose disease and prescribe treatment.

## Maternal Services

Unlike the Frontier Nurses working in the same time period, the BIA nurses only delivered babies in emergencies, when there was no one else to do it.[101] The public health nurses were not certified nurse-midwives, and they worked carefully within their professional boundaries. Rather than delivering patients, the field nurses frequently transported expectant mothers to hospitals. Mollie Reebel reported one case in which she went to extremes to get the patient to the hospital rather than deliver her at home:

> . . . One of the most difficult trips I have ever made was in response to a call about two o'clock one afternoon to go out and see a lady reported as having been in labor for three days with no result. The man who came for me had started before daylight on foot and after reaching the highway had caught a ride. I inquired how far the hogan was, and was assured that it was not very far. Maybe six miles off the highway, and about twelve miles up the highway . . . I took Laura Sherman with me for interpreter and with the Indian man as guide, we started out. After we left the highway we went sixteen miles. Again over places where there was not even a wagon road. Found the patient in terrible condition, put her in the car and headed for Ship Rock where we arrived at 7 PM having covered sixty-four miles from Nava. The patient was given immediate attention and is now recovering, so the trip was well worth while. . . . [102]

For the most part, instead of serving as midwives, the BIA nurses worked as public health nurses, teaching expectant and new mothers how to sew layettes for their infants, how to bathe their babies and care for their skin, how to prevent infantile diarrhea (which was prevalent on the reservation), and how to provide a more nutritious diet for their children. The nurses also conducted prenatal clinics and followed mothers and babies after the delivery, frequently treating infected and bleeding umbilical cords.[103]

There was one problem, however—sometimes there was no one else available to deliver babies when they arrive prematurely or precipitously. Mary Zillitas recounted delivering a baby after receiving physician instructions over the telephone,[104] and in her July 1935 report, Nena Seymour documented: "One pre-natal hospitalized and one premature baby delivered."[105] As in other instances, the BIA nurses simply did what they had to do.

## The 1940s

As World War II engulfed America's energy and tapped its resources, less funding was available for the Indian programs. However, the public health services continued, albeit with shortages in personnel, as was true of hospitals and public health agencies across the country.[106]

During the 1940s, advances in medicine brought other changes to the BIA health services. Care of infectious diseases improved as new drugs like the sulfonamides and penicillin became available. Mobile x-ray units were instituted to screen for tuberculosis, and hospitals specializing in the treatment of TB and crippled children were available in Salt Lake City.[107]

Meanwhile, the field nurses were still de facto diagnosing. Whether or not they recognized it themselves, others with whom the nurses worked acted on their diagnoses. BIA nurse Delores Young recounted one instance in which the school superintendent trusted her judgment without question:

> While at Fort Wingate, N.M., a school girl developed abdominal pain about 8 PM one evening. I advised sending her to Fort Defiance Hospital to be checked. The school superintendent called the school driver saying, "We have to take a girl to the hospital. Miss Young says she's got appendicitis."[108]

## The 1950s: The BIA and the
## United States Public Health Service

In 1955, Congress transferred medical care from the BIA to the United States Public Health Service (USPHS). By then, the entire Indian Health Service was more structured. "By 1955, the Bureau had entered into contracts for care of Indians in 65 general community hospitals, 16 tuberculosis hospitals, and 5 mental hospitals. It also was paying for care on a fee basis at more than 180 additional general or specialized non-Indian hospitals." The policy adopted in 1952 was that the Indian Health facilities would be closed whenever "other similar facilities are available to the eligible Indians without segregation. . . ."[109]

Despite the gradual closure of many of the Indian Health facilities, the nurses' work in schools and clinics continued—sometimes in conjunction with hospital or specialty clinic services. In her annual report for March 1955 to July 1956, public health nurse Lillian Watson noted that PPD testing and Mantoux testing of the school children was being done, and those with active TB were "urged to come to the hospital clinic for chest x-rays." She went on to report, "Nursing conferences were utilized not only to give health supervision and to screen the morbidity cases, but at most of them the nurse made it a point to have some planned demonstrations, such as that of preparing powdered milk, care of skin sores and bathing the baby. Although many of the mothers wondered at a nurse's being interested in her 'well' children, they were coming to see the nurses in increasing numbers . . . and they seemed to be beginning to understand what we were trying to do. . . ." Watson also noted that she was able to "assist at the crippled children's clinics held at Tuba City three times a year by Dr. Paul Pemberton from Salt Lake City."[110]

By the 1950s, some of the educational efforts undertaken by the BIA nurses in the 1920s and 1930s were beginning to pay off. In a September 1957 monthly narrative, one nurse (unidentified) reported that the mothers in the Window Rock area had become very "diarrhea-conscious"—aware of the "great killer of Navajo babies."[111] Some things did not change, however. Even with increased funding and a new bureaucratic structure, the field nurses continued to face many of the same challenges they had for decades. As Watson wrote in her 1955 annual report:

> Many problems are here. We have all repeated them many times . . .
> about automobiles not adapted to sand dunes and mud, about our
> moving population, about the distances we travel, about the lack of
> water and sanitary facilities, about our need for more x-ray facilities,
> about our need for [TB] sanitoria right here on the reservation so that

> families can visit . . . about the need for tonsillectomies and hearing
> devices for children . . . and about so many other things we hardly
> know where to stop. . . . [112]

During this period, the nurses continued to hold nursing clinics throughout the reservation—often outdoors. According to Harold Foster, who worked as a chauffeur and interpreter in the 1950s: "We moved our office 5 or 6 times in one year, (no office space) and carried our family records in the car. We had our Nursing conference under a tree or in the back seat of the service car. . . . "[113] Clearly, an underfunded public health service was still a problem. And there were other problems looming for the nurses—these from their own professional organization, the American Nurses Association (ANA). It was midcentury, and the nursing profession, working from a positivistic epistemology, was struggling to define its scientific base and the boundaries of the discipline. So, in 1955, while nurses in the Frontier Nursing Service and the newly formed Indian Health Service were diagnosing patients and initiating treatments either according to "standing orders" or on their own, the American Nurses Association developed a model definition of nursing that would constrain the professional practice of nursing for the next several decades. The definition, published in 1955 and adopted by many states shortly thereafter, emphasized the fact that nurses were neither to diagnose nor prescribe. According to the ANA:

> The practice of professional nursing means the performance for
> compensation of any act in the observation, care and counsel of the
> ill . . . or in the maintenance of health or prevention of illness . . . or
> the administration of medications and treatments as prescribed by a
> licensed physician. . . . *The foregoing shall not be deemed to include acts*
> *of diagnosis or prescription* of therapeutic or corrective measures.[114]
> (emphasis added)

Although the ANA may simply have been seeking clarity in defining the discipline's boundaries, its exclusion of the acts of diagnosis and prescription interrupted nurses' autonomy in practice settings in which they were providing care to those to whom it would otherwise be denied.[115] The ANA's restrictive definition of nursing also set the stage for continued conflicts over the nurses' legal authority to expand their role to include the privilege of making diagnoses and writing prescriptions. These conflicts—between medicine and nursing—would surface in the 1960s with the institution of the nurse-practitioner role in primary care. In the meantime, inside hospitals in the 1950s, other issues were being addressed.

# CHAPTER 5

# Verbal Orders and Hospital Nursing

## Expanding Nurses' Scope of Practice in the Mid-Twentieth Century

### Eliminating Errors in Medication

. . . If by some miracle, I could address a plea to all members of the medical profession who give orders for medications, I should say something like this—"We are neither sentimental about our functions as nurses nor under false impressions concerning our relative responsibilities. We want to carry out your orders because we, like you, desire to help our patients. Sometimes, however, you do make it unnecessarily difficult for us. You insist on our taking verbal orders when we are taught not to do so. You often write orders we can interpret only with great difficulty or not at all, either because you do not write legibly or because your directions are not clear.[1]

Margene O. Faddis, RN, Associate Professor of Nursing

Writing in the *American Journal of Nursing* in 1939, Associate Professor Margene O. Faddis was expressing her concern about medication errors in hospitals. Faddis addressed two of the major problems: (1) physicians were asking general staff nurses to accept "verbal orders" for patient medications rather than writing those orders on the patient's chart, and (2) physicians' written orders were often illegible and incomprehensible. Both concerns were valid. In the 1930s, as in previous decades, nurses were not supposed to accept verbal orders given by physicians. That is, the physician had to see the patient and write the medication order on the chart, rather than simply giving a "verbal" order over the telephone or in a hallway of the hospital. In fact, physicians had to write and sign not only all medication orders, but all other treatment and dietary orders, as well.

Only a small percentage of the nurses working in the United States had the freedom allowed them in practice settings like the Henry Street Settlement, the Frontier Nursing Service, or the Indian Health Service. Even fewer nurses worked as nurse anesthetists. In 1939, more than half of all nurses working in America worked in hospitals.[2] For years, most graduate nurses had worked in private-duty nursing, in patients' homes.[3] Student nurses had staffed the hospitals. With the collapse of the economy in the 1930s, however, many graduates sought hospital employment.

In the hospital, there were no standing orders for nurses to follow in the absence of a physician. Even "p.r.n" orders (*pro-re-nata*—Latin for "as needed") were to be written specifically for each patient. For example, a physician might write on a patient's chart: "Give ASA, grs. 5 prn q4h for pain," meaning that the nurse was permitted to give the patient one aspirin (5 grains) every four hours as was needed to treat pain.

The purpose of having written rather than verbal orders was to prevent errors in the nurse's interpretation of the orders, including specifics concerning for which patient the medication (or diet or activity order) was intended, the exact dose of a medication, or the specific route of administration. If the doctor had not written the order clearly, which was often the case, the nurse could misinterpret it and make a medication error.

Unlike the Visiting Nurses at Henry Street Settlement, nurse anesthetists, Frontier Nurses in Appalachia, and field nurses working for the Bureau of Indian Affairs (later, the Indian Health Service), all of whom had postgraduate training in their specialty (public health, anesthesia nursing, or nurse-midwifery), the majority of hospital staff nurses,[4] also known as "general duty" nurses, did not have additional education after they graduated from nursing school. Most graduated from hospital-based diploma programs, not colleges and universities, and they had been taught only the basics about physiology, pathophysiology, and pharmacology.[5] General staff nurses did not have the advanced education necessary to make in-depth assessments of their patients' signs and symptoms, nor were they expected to.

For a century, physicians had claimed that the acts of diagnosis and prescription were theirs alone; the nursing profession had never challenged that claim. Ever since Florence Nightingale had refused to care for the sick and injured soldiers in the Crimea until she had a specific request or order from the surgeon in charge, the nursing profession had clung to the belief that nurses were to carry out physicians' orders rather than take any initiative in ordering and implementing care. Physicians even ordered diets for patients, an activity that nurses were more informed about and more capable of implementing. For example, one popular 1902 textbook of nursing included an entire chapter on recipes for broths and gruel, as well as the nutritional requirements of patients with specific disease conditions. Nonetheless, the author was adamant that the physician should make dietary decisions for the patient. According to that text: "What kind of food is to be given in each case will usually be decided by the physician; how best to prepare and administer it are matters for the nurse to know."[6] The boundary line between the professions was clear. Nurses made and recorded patient observations; physicians analyzed the data presented to them. Physicians prescribed treatments, dietary therapy, and medicines; nurses carried out orders. State medical practice acts reinforced these divisions.

## Medicine and Nursing in the Early Twentieth Century

Since the founding of the American Medical Association in 1847, allopathic physicians had been working to gain control of medical care in the United States. In the late nineteenth century, scientific advances in surgery and widespread acceptance of the germ theory and antisepsis gave physicians the credibility they wanted. The rise of professional nursing, coupled with hospital reform, changed the reputation of hospitals from almshouses for the poor to places of healing and scientific medical care. The initiation of medical licensure, the revolutionary changes in medical education that occurred after the Flexner report in 1910,[7] new medical technologies such as the x-ray, the electrocardiogram (ECG),[8] and new diagnostic tests such as the complete blood count and urinalysis further increased physicians' control of their profession. According to historians Rosemary Stevens and Joel Howell, the changes and new technologies also increased the public's confidence in doctors and hospitals.[9] By the 1920s, middle-class Americans accepted hospitalization for specific medical interventions that had "highly successful outcomes, particularly: obstetrical deliveries, appendectomies, and tonsillectomies and adenoidectomies."[10] Because of the widespread problem of tuberculosis, Americans also were willing to enter specialized hospitals—sanitariums and preventoriums—for treatment of that disease.

As Michael Bliss and Chris Feudtner have so clearly described, the discovery of insulin in 1922 provided further evidence of the promise of research and physician-prescribed medicines.[11] With the use of sulfa drugs in the 1930s, physicians were demonstrating that they could cure such previously fatal diseases as pneumonia and nephritis (kidney infection).[12] The use of the "miracle drug" penicillin (discovered by Alexander Fleming in 1928 and widely marketed in World War II), medical advances in World War II, and postwar "space-age" medical technology also increased the American public's respect and admiration for the medical profession. The words "physician" and "cure" became synonymous. And, according to his-torians Barbara Melosh and Susan Reverby, although the public respected and trusted nurses (educated in training schools, middle-class, and female), they saw them as the "caring" profession, "hand-maidens" to better-educated, higher-class, male physicians.[13] Even hospital nurses themselves, the majority of whom were students, did little to change this widespread conviction. In fact, they promoted it. Inside hospitals, gradu-ate nurses worked as nursing supervisors, nursing directors, or nurse anes-thetists. Student nurses handled the management of the wards, including bathing and feeding patients, as well as giving treatments and medications ordered by physicians. And the students simply followed orders.

## Following Orders

Thus, by the 1940s, when the majority of graduate nurses had shifted their place of employment from private duty in patients' homes to staff nursing in hospitals,[14] the boundaries of medicine and nursing had been clearly established. Both professions accepted as fact that doctors were responsible for giving medication orders; nurses, both students and grad-uates, followed them. These orders were to be written, not given verbally. According to a 1948 textbook of nursing:

> In all instances the physician is responsible for writing and signing the order for the drug. . . . In extreme emergencies a verbal order may be carried out by the nurse, but this order should later be written and signed by the physician.[15]

Unlike the nurse working in an urban tenement, in an isolated cabin in Appalachia, or in a remote trading post on an Indian reservation, or the nurse anesthetist who had to rely on her own observations to make criti-cal decisions while the surgeon operated, the general staff nurse working on the wards in an American hospital did not need to act on her own accord. Physicians were readily available. Inside the hospital, therefore, there were no "standing orders" to be followed when the physician was not present. Moreover, the bureaucratic system of hospital administration and the hierarchy within nursing—from the staff nurse to the head nurse to the nursing supervisor and finally to the director of nursing, ensured that decision making went up a nursing chain of command.[16]

Nowhere was the chain of command more rigid than it was in the administration of medications. Usually, the head nurse used a "case assign-ment method," in which she assigned each staff nurse to care for a specific number of patients. In this system, each nurse was responsible for her own patients' medications.[17] According to a 1939 *AJN* article:

> Every department . . . has a medicine board. . . . Across the board there are fifteen spaces—twelve for the day hours and three others. There is one for p.r.n. medicines . . . and one for special medications that are not easily classified. . . . As we work on a case assignment method here, each nurse is responsible for her medications and each nurse is required to consult the medicine board before she begins her assignments in the morning. She is responsible for moving her own cards, charting her medicines as given and removing a card . . . when it is not needed. All medicines are listed individually with the name of the patient, room number, medicine, amount and hours to be given.[18]

During the day, if the nurse needed to contact the doctor about a drug order, she would go to the head nurse, who would discuss the issue with the physician. If, however, the nurse needed an order at night, when the head nurse was not available, she would report the need to the nurse in charge of the unit, who would in turn call the nursing supervisor. The supervisor would then telephone the physician about the problem.[19] The physician would analyze the information presented and respond with orders for treatment, giving verbal orders to the nurse supervisor (whom he trusted) over the telephone, and signing them in the morning. If the situation warranted, the physician might come into the hospital to see the patient in person.

The process took time. Moreover, the reality was that the staff nurse was the first to assess the patient's problem. She was the one who was present at the bedside, and she had been trained to observe for certain signs and symptoms that indicated critical changes in the patient. Based on her findings, the nurse presented an account of the patient's condition to the nurses above her in the chain of command. Eventually, the facts reached the physician. Nurses soon learned that the way in which signs and symptoms were presented could lead the head nurse or supervisor, and subsequently the physician, to a particular diagnosis and treatment conclusion. So, frequently it was the nurse who clustered symptoms to lead the physician to reach the same conclusion she had already reached. It was a game in some respects, with neither nurse nor physician acknowledging what was going on.[20] According to state medical practice acts, only physicians could diagnose and treat. Certain tasks belonged to physicians, and others to nurses.

What was also unacknowledged was the fact that the boundaries between the two professions had been fluid since the inception of professional nursing. These boundaries would continue to shift as physicians transferred increasing

numbers of responsibilities to nurses. By the mid-twentieth century, the con-
fluence of many social, political, and economic factors, including postwar
hospital reconstruction, increasing life expectancy, the national problem of
heart disease, emerging ideas in patient care delivery, medical specialization,
and advances in medicine and technology would transform medical and
nursing practice.

## Post-World War II Hospital Reconstruction

Immediately after World War II, in 1946, Congress passed the Hospital
Survey and Construction Act (also known as "The Hill Burton Act"), providing large scale funding to modernize aging hospitals and build new ones.
Across the country, hospital administrators seized the opportunity to expand
and renovate their facilities, and by the early 1950s, many hospitals were
under construction. These modern hospitals eliminated the large, open wards
in which nurses could readily observe patients and easily move between beds.
Instead, the renovated hospitals had long halls with numerous private and
semiprivate rooms. Although pleasing to middle-class patients who demanded privacy, the newly configured and expanded hospital spaces, along with the
rising acuity of illness in patients, changed the way in which nurses worked.[21]

In the newly renovated spaces, nurses could neither see the patients
from the nursing station nor observe them when they were busy caring for
a patient in another room. The nurses also had to walk long distances up
and down the hallways to reach patients, and the way in which care had
previously been given to the sickest patients in the ward could no longer
be done. Previously, if a patient needed close observation, the nurses
would move him or her to the front of the ward, near the nurses' desk,
where he or she was always in view. With long halls, and private rooms,
this solution was no longer viable. A logical next step might have been to
assign one nurse to "special" the sickest patient. However, because of
increased patient demand for hospital care and the return of women to the
home after World War II, fewer nurses were working. There were simply
not enough nurses to go around.

Thus, the modern hospitals, coupled with the nursing shortage, demanded a new system of care. Nurse leader Eleanor Lambertson took an interest in
the problem and initiated "team nursing," a task-oriented approach to providing nursing care. In this system, the nursing unit was divided into two or three
nursing teams—each team delivered nursing care to a group of patients, who
were assigned to team members according to the complexity of the patient's
needs. Using this system, licensed practical nurses (LPNs) and nurse's aides
provided direct patient care. Registered nurses served as head nurses, supervi-

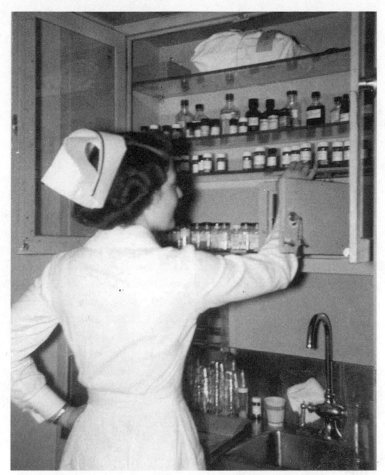

Figure 5.1: RN selecting medications. Joan Lynaugh Collection, Center for the Study of the History of Nursing, University of Pennsylvania

sors, and team leaders,[22] positions that forced the RNs to spend much of their time away from the bedside, preparing assignments, scheduling LPNs and aides, and performing other administrative paperwork. Moreover, the team concept affected the way in which medications were given.

## Passing Meds

One member of each team, usually a graduate RN or a senior student, gave medicines to all of the patients of that team, in most cases half of a large nursing unit of 45 to 60 patients. The procedure for "passing meds," as nurses referred to it, was straightforward. That process, however, involved numerous steps.[23] First, the head nurse transcribed physician orders from the chart to small medicine tickets. Using these medicine tickets, the medication nurse would pour the prescribed drugs from large bottles into small medicine cups, arranging them on a tray.

The tray contained rows of small glass cups, each identified by the medicine ticket on which was written the patient's name, the name of the drug, the method of administration, the bed or room number, and the dose to be given.

The medication nurse would distribute drugs all day, beginning with drugs like insulin that had to be given early in the morning, before breakfast. She then administered the preoperative medications for those patients needing sedation prior to surgery, followed by those medications that were ordered to be given at four-hour intervals, starting at 10:00 AM. Passing medications for an entire team was a challenge, as there were often twenty-two to thirty patients for whom the nurse was responsible. Keeping up with the new drugs that were being prescribed was also an uphill struggle. Counting narcotics and keeping them under lock and key complicated the nurses' work even further.

Few nurses acknowledged to themselves or others that they did indeed know a great deal about the drugs they administered. They had to. According to one 1955 textbook of nursing:

> Giving drugs is one of the nurse's most serious duties. . . . She must know about many drugs and in giving these must be able to follow many physicians' plan of therapy for many patients. . . . It is desirable, therefore that the nurse know the nature of the drug; its local and systemic action and something of the physiological explanation; why the drug is ordered in each case and the result the physician hopes to get; the signs of the intended effect; and the signs of an overdose or of a cumulative toxic effect, or indications that the patient has an idiosyncrasy to the drug. . . . Nurses should know how age, sex, body weight, and time of administration affect the dose. She should know how drugs are excreted . . . for example, the kidneys are irritated by mercury, arsenic, and the sulfa drugs. While the physician is primarily responsible for ordering the medication in the correct dosage, he, being human and often overworked, is subject to error. Lives have been saved by nurses who have recognized mistakes in written orders for drugs. . . . Moreover, a nurse can be successfully prosecuted for carrying out a doctor's order for the wrong drug or a toxic dose, if the court is persuaded that the preparation of the nurse qualified her to recognize the danger of the drug or the dosage.[24]

In other words, even the general duty staff nurse, without training in pharmacotherapeutics, had to know almost as much as physicians did about the medications they gave. Furthermore, they were accountable under their own licenses for the judgments they made.

## Increases in Life Expectancy and Chronic Disease

While hospitals were growing and changing, major changes were occurring in relation to the public's health, medical science and technology, and society. These changes would intersect to create a paradigm shift in the way in which hospitals and nurses delivered care.[25] On the positive side, because of the success of scientific advances in medicine, child and infant mortality rates were declining. Antibiotics, like sulfa drugs and penicillin, did more than provide symptomatic relief; they cured infections.[26] Other illnesses, like polio and tuberculosis, were under investigation, and both vaccine trials and the creation of new drugs were underway. Scientists had developed new machines and medical treatments to diagnose disease and cure patients, including the electrocardiogram (ECG), chest x-ray, urinalysis, and blood work.[27] Americans were living longer. Between 1940 and 1950, the average life expectancy rose 4.4 years for white men (to 66.5 years) and 6.4 years for white women (to 72.2 years).[28] On the negative side, despite these innovations, chronic illnesses, like cancer, stroke, and heart disease, were emerging as the major problems facing Americans. Of these, heart disease—soon known as "the coronary problem"—was the number one killer.

## The "Coronary Problem"

The "Coronary Problem" in post–World War II America was a significant one. As President Harry S. Truman noted in his 1949 address to the nation, "The tremendous toll of the heart diseases must be of deep concern to all our citizens. Combating the nation's leading cause of death has become our most serious national health problem. . . . The heart diseases, I am informed, now account for one out of every two deaths after the age of forty."[29]

Those dying were typically white males in their mid-forties and fifties. Many "dropped dead" outside of the hospital before they could reach care. Those who managed to stay alive long enough to reach the hospital were often placed in the new private rooms to ensure quiet and rest, visited only every few hours by the medication nurse or the LPN or aide assigned to check their blood pressure, pulse, and temperature. Close to 40 percent died without warning from sudden cardiac arrest—alone in their private rooms.[30]

For the remaining 60 percent who survived the first few days after a heart attack (myocardial infarction, or MI), new therapies offered hope for survival. The radiological technique of cardiac catheterization offered promise for the diagnosis of blocked coronary arteries. Once diagnosed, these blocked arteries could be "bypassed" with veins harvested from the patient's own legs in open-heart surgery—made possible by new cardiopulmonary bypass technology in the 1950s.[31] Those who did not need surgery might benefit from recently invented, high-tech cardiac pacemakers. Others could receive cardiac drugs such as quinidine gluconate, potassium salts, and procainamide hydrochloride (Procainamide) and Lanatoside C (for rapid intravenous digitalization to strengthen the heart beat) that were used to treat atrial and ventricular arrhythmias.[32]

Meanwhile, reports of the success of external cardiopulmonary resuscitation (CPR) and external cardiac defibrillation in saving lives after cardiac arrest filled the medical literature. Perhaps more patients could be saved.

Despite the new treatments and drugs, mortality from heart attacks remained high, and the nation was concerned. For the most part, the patients dying from acute myocardial infarction were white, middle-class men in the prime of life who played an important role in the American economy. Moreover, they included prominent national leaders whose medical conditions attracted national press coverage. In July 1955, Senate Majority Leader Lyndon Baines Johnson (LBJ) experienced a massive heart attack.[33] Johnson remained in the US Naval Hospital in Bethesda for six weeks, during which time members of the press were in constant attendance. Only two months later, on September 24, 1955, President Dwight D. Eisenhower suffered a coronary thrombosis.[34] The press coverage of the president's illness was immediate and continued throughout his seven-week stay at Fitzsimmons Army Hospital and subsequent convalescence at home.[35] Heart disease had the nation's attention. It also had the attention of the middle-aged white male legislators who made up Congress. It would not be long before they appropriated federal funds to address the problem.

## Emerging Ideas in Patient Care Delivery Systems

While the nation focused on the larger problem of what to do about heart disease, inside hospitals across the nation nurses were struggling to care for coronary and other critically ill patients in the newly configured environment. The sickest patients needed constant observation and care, even when they were in private rooms at some distance from the nurses' station. The patient who could afford to do so hired a private-duty nurse to stay in his room. For the patient who could not afford a private nurse, the head nurse tried to move him to a room nearer the nursing station. The solution worked for acutely ill trauma or surgical patients who needed nursing treatments at frequent intervals. However, the solution did not work for cardiac patients. The heart patient needed rest in a quiet environment, and the rooms nearest the station were not quiet. On the other hand, the rooms that provided peace and quiet also provided a setting in which sudden death could occur unobserved. Something had to be done, and that something would have profound implications for nurses' scope of practice.

In 1957, Faye Abdellah and her colleague Josephine Starchan, both nurses at Manchester Memorial Hospital in Connecticut, attempted to find a solution. Together, they proposed a system of "Progressive Patient Care," defining it as the "organization of facilities, services and staff around the medical and nursing needs of the patient."[36] In this system, patients would progress from special care units where they stayed when they were critically ill, to "step-down units," and on to "home care." To test the idea, Abdellah and Starchan established a special care unit at Manchester Memorial and equipped the twenty-seven bed unit with routine and emergency supplies, including oxygen tents, suctioning equipment, and emergency drugs. The unit would be used for "those patients who were critically ill or in need of very close nursing observation and attention."[37] Patients with acute cardiac conditions met the requirement for "close nursing observation" and were admitted to the special care unit. There, nurses were taking on new responsibilities, including the tasks of inserting intravenous (IV) lines and drawing blood specimens,[38] tasks which until the crisis situation of World War II had been done solely by physicians.

According to Abdellah, "Since most emergency situations arise or are cared for on this unit, the nurses need to be especially alert in observing signs and symptoms of possible complications. Technical competence, skill in giving direction and guidance to team members, and the physical, mental, and emotional ability to meet day-by-day crises are essential."[39] Meeting the "day-by-day" crises would soon mean that a nurse had to give emergency cardiac drugs intravenously—in some instances without waiting for a physician's written or verbal order.

The idea of progressive patient care, which included step down units, (for the care of patients who were not critically ill) and home care in addition to intensive care, soon had widespread acceptance. Of the three parts, hospital administrators, physicians, and nurses were particularly interested in the concept of intensive care, the most exciting and innovative aspect. As a result, intensive care units opened in hospitals throughout the country in the 1950s and early 1960s. Most were general medical–surgical units, open to patients with a variety of acute illnesses and trauma. Several were designated specifically to house postoperative cardiac surgical patients. Very few admitted patients who had had a heart attack. These patients were assigned to quiet, private rooms on a general nursing unit.

## Advances in Medical Science and Technology

Advances in medical science and technology continued after World War II. In 1959, Drs. William B. Kouwenhoven, James Jude, and G. Guy Knickerbocker at the Johns Hopkins University School of Medicine experimented with dogs and discovered an effective method of "massaging the heart without thoracotomy"—that is, without surgically opening the chest.[40] Two years later, the same research team reported that they had used the method of external cardiac massage on 118 patients, 28 of whom survived to leave the hospital.[41] This dramatic discovery of the effectiveness of external CPR followed on the heels of a series of medical research reports on cardiac defibrillation. In 1941, Dr. Claude Beck, a surgeon at Case Western Reserve School of Medicine in Cleveland, Ohio had reported the first two attempts of cardiac defibrillation during surgery. His conclusion, that "the heart can be defibrillated . . . a coordinated beat can be restored,"[42] had been ground breaking. When they published again in 1956, Beck and his colleagues emphasized the necessity of having an electrocardiogram (ECG) convey data about the electrical activity of the heart. That way, the physician could know whether the underlying cardiac mechanism responsible for the death was cardiac arrest (flat line) or a fatal arrhythmia (electrical irregularity). According to the researchers:

> Since cardiac arrhythmias cannot be diagnosed by inspection alone, easy access to an electrocardiograph is necessary. Precise knowledge of the cardiac mechanism is of utmost importance if successful restoration of a normal rhythm is to be intelligently planned.[43]

That precise identification of the mechanism responsible for cardiac arrest required that the patient would have to be connected to an electrocardiograph machine at all times and that someone with specialized knowledge in interpreting ECGs be present at the bedside when sudden death occurred. Therein lay the problem: cardiac patients were not routinely attached to ECGs. In fact, a nurse would have to locate an electrocardiograph machine and wheel it into the room in an emergency situation.

Furthermore, nurses, who were present in the hospital twenty-four hours a day (if not directly at the bedside), could not interpret the electrocardiograms. Neither could many general practitioners—if and when they arrived at the scene of the emergency and ordered one to be taken.

## Nursing Care of the Patient with a Heart Attack, circa 1950s

Until this time, despite the advances in science and technology, the nurse caring for heart attack patients in the postwar period continued to care for them as she had for years. Her role involved serving as the physicians' eyes and hands, making observations, and collecting physiologic data such as temperature, pulse rate, and blood pressure—tasks that had been delegated to nurses over the first half of the century. In doing so, the nurses used technology that the physician considered to be "easy enough for the nurse to do."[44]

For example, by the 1950s, physicians had delegated to nurses the task of taking blood pressures. To do this, the nurses used blood pressure cuffs and stethoscopes. Stethoscopes, however, were to be used by the nurse only for checking blood pressure. Only physicians were to use the stethoscope to listen to a patient's heart and lung sounds. The nurse, on the other hand, was expected to observe the depth, quality, and rate of respirations and count the pulse at the patient's wrist, noting whether the pulse was strong or weak, bounding or thready, regular or irregular. Well into the 1960s, nurses' notes were typically a litany of facts without analysis. Temperature, pulse and respiration were recorded at specific intervals and graphed once a shift. Nurses did not usually write their analysis of the observations they made. More often, one would have to read between the lines to ascertain what the nurse was thinking, which could be done by the way that she clustered signs and symptoms in her notes. She might, for example, write, "Patient complaining of chest pain. Color: dusky. Skin: cold and clammy. Pulse: thready, rate 100. Also short of breath, respirations 28. BP 80/60. Urinary output declining from 70 cc per hour to 20 cc per hour. Doctor notified." What the nurse meant, of course, was that the patient was failing to maintain an adequate blood pressure; failing to profuse his skin, lungs, and kidneys; and was in all likelihood suffering shock. In the extreme instance of sudden death (as the author recalls) the nurse was only expected to record: "Apneic, pulseless, cyanotic, unresponsive, pupils fixed and dilated. Appears dead. Doctor notified."[45] Indeed, as historian Margarete Sandelowski has argued, nurses were expected to "collect, record, and interpret information vital to the diagnosis—and therefore to the treatment and prognosis . . . without making any claims to participating in diagnosis."[46]

In addition to making and recording observations, the nurse's job for the patient with a heart attack included the traditional tasks of putting the patient to bed and making him or her comfortable. Writing in the *American Journal of Nursing* in 1961, Mildred Crawley, Chief of the Heart Nursing Service, National Institutes of Health, described the nurse's role in the care of the acutely ill cardiac patient:

> During the first hour of a patient's hospitalization, the doctor must make an initial examination, an electrocardiograph will be taken, blood may be drawn for analysis, probably oxygen will be started, and medication will be given for pain. During all these activities, the nurse or aide is expected to admit the patient, care for his belongings, undress him and get him settled as comfortably as possible in bed, [and] care for the needs and questions of the family. . . .[47]

The boundaries between medicine and nursing were clear. The physician would examine the patient. He or a medical student would take the cardiogram and draw blood. Meanwhile, the nurse would settle the patient in bed and put his or her belongings in the bedside table. Then the nurse would take the temperature, pulse, and respirations as ordered and record her observations at the appropriate intervals. Following doctor's orders, she would also give injections of morphine and administer tablets of nitroglycerine "p.r.n." to the patient complaining of chest pain. Or she might ask the medication nurse to administer these drugs. She certainly didn't read the electrocardiogram (if, in fact, it was taken). In the course of the patient's illness, only the physician would diagnose cardiac arrhythmias and decide on the proper treatment.

By the early 1960s, however, it was becoming apparent that these clearly delineated boundaries of medical and nursing practice were not always in the best interest of the patient. Neither was the delay involved in getting an order for an emergency drug or waiting for a busy medication nurse to administer morphine or nitroglycerine to the patient complaining of chest pain. Chest pain was a life-threatening emergency that required immediate diagnosis and treatment. Moreover, the prompt use of new drugs like lidocaine and atropine to treat lethal cardiac arrhythmias could be life saving. Waiting even three minutes for a doctor to arrive at the scene to order these drugs could prove fatal for the patient. The solution was obvious, at least to a handful of physicians scattered around the world.[48] The nurse, present at the bedside twenty-four hours a day, seven days a week, would have to learn from physicians how to diagnose and treat cardiac arrhythmias. She could *not* wait for orders, even if by not doing so, she invaded territory traditionally claimed by the medical profession.

## The Genesis of the CCU: Bethany Hospital, Kansas City

Bethany Hospital in Kansas City, Kansas, was in many ways similar to the 6,000 other community hospitals in America in the 1950s. Like them, Bethany had experienced phenomenal growth, subsidized by Hill Burton funds. In fact, the construction of a large west wing at Bethany in 1957 provided the 90-bed hospital with an additional 110 beds, more than doubling its size. And, like other newly renovated hospitals, instead of the traditional, open wards, Bethany now had long corridors off of which opened multiple private and semiprivate rooms.

The new configuration stressed a system already short of nurses. The arrangement also blocked the nurses' view of critically ill patients. Consequently, patients who needed 24-hour-a-day observation were either placed near the nurses' station or assigned a private-duty nurse. However, private-duty nurses were not assigned to care for cardiac patients who were considered to be in stable condition. Instead, the hemodynamically stable patient recuperating from a heart attack was often assigned to a private room near the end of a hall, where he could rest quietly. A nurse would check him periodically, most often when she was passing medications. Aides would take his blood pressure and pulse at regular intervals, usually every four hours; however, even stable, pain-free cardiac patients were dying suddenly and without warning. At Bethany, the mortality rate from a heart attack (myocardial infarction) was 35 percent.[49]

Dr. Hughes W. Day, a 46-year-old internist at Bethany, was concerned about the sudden deaths of his middle-aged cardiac patients. He had also read the medical literature on Dr. Claude Beck's cutting-edge research on cardiac defibrillation. In an attempt to keep his cardiac patients alive, Day initiated a new procedure, calling it "Code Blue."[50] According to his protocol, when a nurse discovered a patient who had no pulse or respirations, she was to call the hospital switchboard operator and ask her to announce "Code Blue" over the hospitals' loudspeaker. The call would alert a special team of physicians and nurses to respond to these cardiac emergencies. The idea was an excellent one—at least in theory. In reality, the success of the Code Blue protocol at Bethany was less than optimal.

There were several problems. First, there was no effective alarm system to alert the nurses that a patient had suffered sudden cardiac arrest. Patients died quietly in their rooms. If, by chance, the nurse did discover that a patient had suddenly stopped breathing and/or had no pulse, the RN had to call the code and get the code cart to the patient's room. Doctors then had to respond from wherever they were in the hospital. Precious minutes were wasted. Often, it was too late to save the patient, who by that time had significant brain damage owing to lack of oxygen.

The nurses and doctors used the protocol for about ten months without success. There was no change in mortality statistics for patients who suffered cardiac or pulmonary arrest—of those in whom resuscitation was attempted, only 4 percent survived.[51]

Frustrated by the poor success rates of the Code Blue procedure, Day decided to try a new approach. He would electronically monitor all cardiac patients, leaving the cardiac monitor outside the patient's room in the hall with the arrhythmia alarms set. If the heart rate was too high or too low, the alarms would sound. That way, *theoretically,* the nurse caring for the patient could immediately observe an arrhythmia or respond to alarms signifying cardiac arrest or changes in heart rate. Again the reality was quite different. As Judith Stuart, a Bethany nurse in 1961, recalled:

> One of the engineers at Bethany, Johnny Walker, rigged up a cardiac monitor for Dr. Day. Originally the cardiac patients were just put in a room out on the floor and hooked to a monitor that sat outside the room. When the patient's heart stopped, the alarm would go off and the nurse would call Dr. Day at home so he could come to the hospital and try to resuscitate the patient. Usually it was too late because more than ten minutes had elapsed.[52]

It was becoming apparent that the electronic equipment that Day had installed could not be used to its fullest capacity without specially trained nurses who could operate it effectively and interpret the arrhythmias—essentially nurses who could diagnose.

Having reached this conclusion, Day collaborated with hospital administrator Walter Coburn and requested funding from the John A. Hartford Foundation, proposing to develop a cardiac unit in which specially trained nurses could provide care for cardiac patients. Day proposed that the coronary unit be attached to an intensive care unit already being planned. That way, nurses who were experienced in caring for critically ill patients would be available to help out in the coronary section during emergencies. Each cardiac patient would be continuously monitored on an electrocardiograph machine. Day himself would teach the nurses how to interpret the printouts from that machine, telling them what to look for and what to report to him. He would also teach them about the emergency drugs used to treat arrhythmias. The idea sold to the Hartford Foundation, and the Hartford Intensive Coronary Care Unit, with its seven intensive care beds and its four beds for coronary patients, opened on May 20, 1962.[53] Almost simultaneously, Lawrence E. Meltzer, MD, conducted a similar experiment in the Presbyterian Hospital in Philadelphia.

## The Presbyterian Nursing Experiment

Apparently unaware of the work of Hughes Day in Kansas City, Lawrence E. Meltzer, a seasoned research physician at Presbyterian Hospital in Philadelphia, applied to the Division of Nursing, United States Public Health Service (USPHS) in 1962, requesting funding for a research project in the newly established cardiac research unit at Presbyterian. Working with the chief of cardiology, J. Roderick Kitchell, MD, Meltzer proposed a nurse-focused study in Presbyterian's recently completed, two-bed cardiac unit to see if monitoring and intervention by specially trained nurses could reduce the high incidence of sudden cardiac deaths.[54]

Like Hughes Day at Bethany, Lawrence Meltzer was determined to find a way to reduce the high mortality after heart attacks—even if it meant delegating new responsibilities to nurses. Hypothesizing that he could prevent the sudden and unexpected deaths by electrical cardiac monitoring,[55] Meltzer proposed to use a "specially trained team of nurses, cardiologists and resident physicians functioning in a hospital unit planned solely for the treatment of acute myocardial infarction [heart attack] in which patients would be monitored by ECG and have all necessary equipment available to interrupt would-be catastrophic arrhythmias," including intravenous drugs.[56] The proposed team would include registered nurses who had specific skills in caring for cardiac patients. These nurses would assume a responsibility previously assumed only by research cardiologists or anesthetists: they would interpret the heart rhythms displayed on the cardiac monitors and initiate emergency treatment for life-threatening arrhythmias. In fact, they would defibrillate patients, start intravenous lines, give oxygen, and treat cardiac arrhythmias with various drugs according to "standing orders" left by the physician. According to Meltzer's proposal, "the nurse, by definition of her responsibility, will be the vital member of the scientific team."[57]

Based on this new role, Meltzer predicted that the coronary care nurses' status within the profession would be affected. According to Meltzer, "If nurses are capable of performing these exacting tasks and assuming this degree of responsibility, the role of the nurse will be materially different than her present day status."[58] As he would later write in the preface to his book, *Intensive Care: A Manual for Nurses,* "it was apparent that a separate, higher division within the nursing profession must be established for this purpose in the form of nurse specialists."[59]

## Creating Specific Knowledge for Nurses

The key to the entire coronary care project was, by necessity, the nurses' advanced training in the highly specialized area of coronary care. According to Presbyterian CCU's nursing director Rose Pinneo, "It became obvious that specialized training beyond basic nursing education was essential in order for nurses to fulfill their role in the coronary care unit."[60] Meltzer was at first of the opinion that this specialized training should include complex knowledge of twelve-lead electrocardiograms (the view of the electrical activity of the heart from twelve different perspectives), but he later decided that the nurses needed to learn to interpret only one of the "views," that from lead II, one that clearly showed the cardiac rhythm. He also thought that they should know principles of cardiology, pared down to the essential knowledge needed for safe practice. In Meltzer's opinion, the nurses needed to learn to recognize the patterns of the basic cardiac arrhythmias and identify those that were life-threatening. In addition, they needed to know the drugs to be used to treat the arrhythmias and how to defibrillate patients.[61]

After the brief introductory course and a few weeks of orientation to the monitoring equipment and the unit procedures, the CCU nurses learned on the job, practicing their newly acquired skills as they cared for patients. Organized clinical conferences occasionally supplemented nurse-to-nurse or physician-to-nurse training. Every month or so, Meltzer met with the nurses and reviewed cases in which the patient had had a cardiac arrest, and he "would point out areas in which the nurses might have done something different."[62] With Meltzer's help, the novice coronary care nurses gained specialized knowledge so they could take on the new responsibilities of caring for critically ill patients who had suffered heart attacks. Whether or not their new responsibilities were within the legal scope of practice was a separate issue, but one that would quickly rise to the surface in medical and nursing discussions.

## Standing Orders

In addition to the cardiac monitoring and emergency cardiopulmonary resuscitation and defibrillation, CCU nurses also assumed other tasks formerly performed by physicians. Some of the responsibilities were documented in a standing order set—a list of medical procedures and "p.r.n." medications written ahead of time to cover foreseeable circumstances in which the nurse might have to initiate treatment in the absence of a physician. Based on these standing orders, nurses attached patients to electrocardiograph machines, inserted intravenous lines to provide fluids, performed venipunctures to draw blood samples, administered oxygen, and gave emergency medications like intravenous morphine, quinidine, lidocaine, dilantin, or sublingual nitroglycerine. In addition, they conducted ongoing physical assessments of the patient's condition.[63] In a 1965 speech, nurse director Rose Pinneo described the nurse's role during the process of admitting a patient to the coronary care unit:

> Mr. J., a 75-year-old man, was brought to the coronary care unit after a myocardial infarction attack at home. He was dyspneic [short of breath] on admission and had severe chest pain accompanied by anxiety. In evaluating Mr. J., while making him comfortable, the nurse realized that his chest pain must be relieved before she proceeded with any other measures. Therefore, she administered an ordered narcotic. Since dyspnea was another obvious problem, she started oxygen therapy by nasal cannula and evaluated its effectiveness. . . . As soon as possible, she applied chest electrodes and connected them by wires to cardiac monitors. . . . [64]

## After Midnight

The coronary care nurse's role expanded even more after midnight. Defibrillating patients was a classic example. During the day and in the evening, there was usually a physician available who could defibrillate a patient whose cardiac rhythm had degenerated to ventricular fibrillation. After midnight, defibrillating a patient was often up to the nurse. Presbyterian Hospital did have interns and residents on call during the night; however, they did not sleep in the CCU but "catnapped wherever they could find an empty bed. Sometimes this was in the intensive care unit, and sometimes in a bed across the hall from the CCU."[65] As a result, there was often a delay in the resident's arrival in the unit in response to a code. According to coronary care nurse Lynn Warner: "I defibrillated many patients. I worked at night of course, so I was there first."[66] Head nurse Janice Lufkin agreed, noting: "mostly I defibrillated at night when no one was there right away. Sometimes the doctor was away from the unit, in the ER admitting a patient or in the ICU."[67]

Even when the resident or intern was present, the nurse might have to take the lead in treating the patient, as some of the coronary care nurses soon knew more than the house staff about the interpretation of cardiac arrhythmias and the necessary treatments. As Janice Lufkin recalled:

> We soon got experience with the rhythm strips. The interns would even come up the stairs from the ER and ask if we could read the

rhythm strip of an ER patient or interpret their EKG [*sic*]. They would ask if they should admit the patient. We were good at the rhythms, but just OK with the 12 lead EKGs. We could recognize the basics, like ST elevation in some leads . . . the obvious MI. And then we would tell them what to do.[68]

Sometimes the house staff's inexperience was a problem. Coronary care nurse Lynn Warner recalled one instance: "We were giving Dilantin IV for ventricular tachycardia. . . . [T]he residents would try to help, but they would forget to use Normal Saline to mix it in, and the medications would precipitate in the IV line."[69]

By 1970, Meltzer did not mince words when discussing the relationship between house staff and CCU nurses, writing: "The unique role of the CCU nurse and her status on the team should be carefully explained to the house staff. As might be anticipated, the traditional physician-nurse relationship may become distorted in this setting when the nurse is assuming duties and responsibilities beyond those generally expected of nurses . . . the wise house officer will recognize their judgment and expertise."[70]

## An Expanded Role for Nursing

The new environment, with its high-tech equipment, combined with the expectations outlined in Meltzer's research project, demanded that the nurses expand their traditional role. In the early days of the unit's existence, the primary purpose of the CCU project was to determine if the nurses' immediate response to medical emergencies, particularly cardiac arrest, could save lives. Since each minute of delay could be life-threatening, autonomy in decision making during those emergencies was essential. So was the authority to treat the patient. As Pinneo would later explain:

> Utilizing this unique combination of clinical assessment and cardiac monitoring, the nurse makes independent decisions. She determines those situations requiring her immediate intervention to save life prior to the physician's arrival or those situations that warrant calling the physician and waiting for his evaluation. It is in these precious moments that the patient's life may literally be in the hands of the nurse.[71]

What was new was the fact that nurses had to move from simply collecting data and reporting their findings, as they had long been doing when they took temperatures and blood pressures, to interpreting those data and acting on their own assessment when necessary, prior to reporting it to a

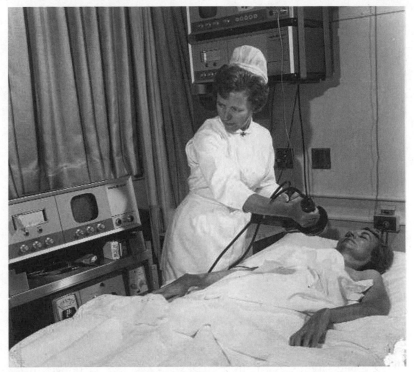

Figure 5.2: Rose Pinneo, RN defibrillating patient. PC, CNHI

physician. The results were impressive—at least at first. Day's success in reducing mortality from sudden death from 43 percent in 1963 (on general hospital units) to 19 percent in the coronary care unit in 1965 received world-wide attention.[72] Meltzer's statistics were similar.[73] Physicians and nurses from all over the world visited Bethany Hospital and Presbyterian Hospital to see for themselves the way that care was implemented in the CCU. The American Heart Association and the American College of Cardiology held national conferences on the topic, attracting hundreds of nurses and cardiologists from around the world. With financial support from the federal government's Regional Medical Programs initiated by President Lyndon B. Johnson in 1965 (P.L. 89–239),[74] coronary care units sprang up around the country. The idea had taken hold. Call nurses had an expanded role within hospitals, and no one was questioning their new responsibilities. Meltzer clearly understood the implications of extending the nurse's role. Discussing the change in 1972, he identified it as critical to the new "scientific team approach," noting, "That the physician delegates unusual authority to the nurse in this team approach . . . is one of the most distinguishing characteristics of the system of intensive coronary care."[75]

## The Blurry Line

These first units were as much an experiment on nurses—to see if they could assume a new role—as they were about decreasing mortality in MI patients. The experiment about nurses' roles was a success. It was apparent that nurses could and would learn new skills and expand their scope of practice. They could also learn medical information, be assertive, make critical decisions at the bedside, and take responsibility for their actions. In doing so, they did, in fact, elevate their status from physician's hand-maiden to emerging nurse specialists. But, despite claims of collegial status in the literature, and despite the fact that the nurses were indeed members of the scientific team, they were not really "equals." Their gender (mostly female), age (twenty-something), educational level (usually diploma education rather than college and postgraduate training), and socioeconomic status as nurses would influence physicians' ability to accept them as colleagues. Nonetheless, the professional relationship between CCU nurses and physicians was quite different in some respects from the traditional nurse/physician relationship. Simply put, the physicians trusted them. These young nurses made independent clinical assessments and treatment decisions in emergency situations. They experienced a new level of autonomy and gained a new level of respect. If the physicians did not like the nurses' new role, they either did not express their feelings or perhaps only discussed it in private with their colleagues. The nurses reported no problems, and in fact, they felt that the new role was well received.[76]

Some aspects of their role did not change, however. The boundary lines between medicine and nursing remained blurry. Even though the nurses worked from standing order sets, and even though they assessed patients, diagnosed such problems as cardiac arrhythmias, heart failure, and cardiogenic shock and selected the appropriate treatment, nurses did not have the legal authority to prescribe medications. Instead, during the night they wrote "verbal orders" (usually given by themselves) for medications and implemented them. The doctors signed the orders when they made rounds in the morning.[77] Nurses negotiated the boundaries of their practice with each individual physician with whom they worked.[78]

Undeniably, with the implementation of the cutting-edge technology and the new knowledge came the shift in responsibilities for nursing that expanded the boundaries of what was considered within their scope of practice. Often the nurses were working outside their legal scope of practice. The shift in boundaries and legal coverage occurred gradually and unsteadily as the decade of the 1960s progressed. Conflicting expectations coincided, as new duties were combined with traditional ones. Coronary care nurses who still needed a physician's order for aspirin or a specific diet for their post-MI patients were entrusted with the authority to identify a fatal cardiac arrhythmia and administer a life-saving cardiac medicine intravenously. On the other hand, the staff nurse who had never before dared call a physician directly was now not only calling him, but was reporting that she had given intravenous atropine, defibrillated his patient, or given an intravenous bolus of lidocaine. Nurses who had been "ordered to care"[79] now stepped over the nursing practice domain line into the realm of scientific medicine, diagnosed arrhythmias, and initiated treatments in dramatic life-saving moments.

## A New Era

Coronary care unleashed a new era for nurses, as the changes that occurred in practice set the stage for the establishment of a collegial relationship between nurses and physicians. In fact, physician-nurse collaborative practice became the norm in these units. Teamwork was essential to the unit's success, and boundaries between the disciplines blurred as a new respect for each other's skills developed. According to historians Fairman and Lynaugh, "Most importantly, nurses and physicians learned to trust each other as they practiced in their own areas of expertise"[80]

The problem was that some of coronary care nursing practice was technically outside of the scope of practice for nursing. Only eight years earlier, the American Nurses Association (ANA) had written the definition of nursing that specifically excluded the acts of diagnosis and prescription. Now, nurses were diagnosing arrhythmias, heart failure, shock, and even death. Whether or not they were "practicing medicine without a license," all depended on how the terms "diagnose" and "prescribe" were defined. Was diagnosing an arrhythmia really medical diagnosis, or was the arrhythmia to be considered a complication of the diagnosis of acute myocardial infarction? What about heart failure or shock? Were they diagnoses or reactions to the myocardial infarction? Was writing a verbal order (from oneself) the same as prescribing? (After all, there was no prescription pad involved.) Or was it simply "furnishing" according to protocols that would have been written had the idea of having such protocols for all possible conditions been considered?[81]

Organized nursing could not agree. Many nursing professors, concerned about carving out a specific role for nurses to separate the profession from medicine, worried that nursing was taking on too many tasks that physicians didn't want to do anymore. However, while the professors, theorists, and other leaders argued over whether nurses should start intravenous lines, defibrillate, draw blood, read electrocardiograms, and so on, the coronary care nurses did what they believed was necessary to save lives. Once again, as had happened in Henry Street, in the field of anesthesia, in the Frontier Nursing Service, and in the Indian Health Service, the realities of practice preceded the legal and professional changes in scope of nursing practice that would be necessary.

The coronary care nurse's work also initiated other practice questions for the profession. If specially trained nurses could diagnose and treat life-threatening arrhythmias in coronary care units, why couldn't specially trained nurses in pediatrics diagnose and treat a child's sore throat or ear infection? If intensive care nurses could use a stethoscope to listen to a patient's heart and lungs in high-tech urban, academic medical centers where doctors were readily available, why couldn't a nurse use a stethoscope to examine a patient in a remote area clinic? And if a nurse could use a stethoscope to listen to a heart, why not an otoscope to look in a patient's ear? Who owned the technology?[82]

The extent of what nurses might learn was also questioned. If the nurse could interpret part of an ECG (one lead) couldn't she learn to interpret the entire twelve-lead ECG? If she could interpret cardiograms, why not interpret x-rays? If she could interpret the results of a blood test to see if the cardiac patient needed more potassium, why couldn't she check the white blood count to see if the patient had an infection? And, if she could learn advanced pharmacology about *cardiac* drugs, couldn't she learn advanced pharmacotherapeutics for a wide variety of drugs?

Moreover, the extent of nurses' authority to furnish and prescribe drugs was an issue. If a nurse could write verbal orders for life-saving intravenous drugs like lidocaine and atropine, couldn't she write a prescription for penicillin, trisulfite pills, or cough medicines like elixir of terpin hydrate—drugs with far less risk to the patient—drugs that nurses had been furnishing for over thirty years in the Frontier Nursing Service and under the Bureau of Indian Affairs? Furthermore, if nurses were capable of taking care of a critically ill patient in intensive care, couldn't they be trusted to manage the care of well babies in collaboration with a physician partner— a job they had been doing for quite some time in the Frontier Nursing Service and in the Indian Health Service? Some thinking along these lines was apparently what Loretta Ford, RN, and Henry Silver, MD, were doing in Colorado in 1965 when they initiated the role of the pediatric nurse-practitioner—a role that would transform graduate education and practice in nursing in the decades to follow—a role that would bring the issue of prescriptive privileges for nurse practitioners to the forefront of debate.

CHAPTER 6

# Nurse Practitioners and the Prescription Pad, 1965–1980

This was what I had been waiting for, the chance to return to my birthplace and work among my people. . . . It was a challenge—one I wanted to be prepared for—and as a condition of acceptance, I asked to be sent for pediatric nurse practitioner training at the University of Colorado Medical Center. The four-month intensive course gave me skills and knowledge which proved a tremendous help in managing conditions for patients of all age groups on the reservation.

Lorraine M. Durran, RN, PNP, Indian Health Service[1]

Pediatric nurse practitioner Lorraine M. Durran, an Indian by birth, was describing the opportunity presented to her in 1970. Her mother, who had been in charge of the Indian Health Service (IHS) health center on the Southern Ute Reservation in Colorado, had just retired. For Lorraine Durran, it was her chance to "make life better" for her people.[2] Her Navajo father had worked with the Bureau of Indian Affairs, and Durran had grown up in Gallup, New Mexico, near the Navajo Reservation. Durran was familiar with the Indians' poverty and poor health, and as a teenager she had been determined to become a nurse. After graduating from a government boarding school and then the University of Colorado School of Nursing, Durran had joined the Colorado Department of Health as a public health nurse in 1967. When she was assigned to work with the Navajos in Shiprock, New Mexico, Durran again realized the Indians' desperate need for early preventive care, particularly noticing that numerous clinics were cancelled because of the "dwindling number of doctors" in the Navajo region.[3] According to her, "My visits to patients' homes, where I recognized health problems and had definite ideas on how they should be managed, reinforced my conviction that the nurse was an untapped resource for the physician-short Federal agency."[4]

Durran was also aware that she needed more than her bachelor's degree in nursing if she were to be adequately prepared to care for patients in the remote desert region. So, when faced with the opportunity to succeed her mother as head of the IHS clinic on the Southern Ute reservation in 1970, she requested nurse-practitioner training at the University of Colorado Medical Center. It was an excellent choice.

The four-month-long program had been in existence since 1965, when assistant professor of nursing Loretta Ford and pediatrician Henry Silver opened it, seeking "to bridge the gap between health care needs of children and families' ability to access and afford primary health care."[5] Their intent was to educate graduate pediatric nurses to provide health care services in rural clinics, essentially expanding the nurse's role in well-child care.[6] According to Ford, an experienced public health nurse who served as the co-director of the project, "I was well aware of the unmet health needs of people of all ages in the community and confident that nurses could be prepared to meet those needs by facilitating access and promoting continuity and coordination of care."[7]

The demonstration project, the first of its kind, was funded by the Commonwealth Foundation and was designed to prepare professional nurses to provide comprehensive well-child care and to manage common childhood health problems. The idea was that the nurse practitioner (NP) would work in a collaborative, collegial relationship with the physicians, not as a physician substitute.[8] The program, which certified RNs as pediatric nurse practitioners (PNPs) without requiring a master's degree, emphasized health promotion and the inclusion of the family in pediatric care.

The Colorado PNP curriculum prepared Durran for the various clinical procedures she would need to perform when she saw patients on her own in the field or when she worked alongside physicians in a clinic. Nurse-practitioner students learned to take health histories and complete physical examinations. They also learned how to devise a list of differential diagnoses and to order laboratory tests, x-rays, and electrocardiograms (ECGs) to "rule out" certain conditions in order to determine a diagnosis. Based on their assessments, PNPs made treatment plans that included medicines.

Pediatric nurse practitioners were to work with physician supervision. In Durran's case, Indian Health Services' (IHS) contract physicians David Grenoble, MD, and Chester Wigton, MD, served as her backup. She could also call Frederick Pintz, MD, the IHS director of the Sante Fe unit, for consultation. According to Durran, she was also given "wide latitude in making referrals to specialists in Durango."[9]

## Specialization and the Shortage of "General Practice" Physicians

Pediatric nurse practitioners' skills could be used in a variety of settings, not only on Indian reservations. PNPs were prepared to work in any pediatric practice; however, the original intent of the Colorado program was to prepare NPs to work in underserved rural areas of the country. There were simply not enough general practice physicians in the country, and they were especially scarce in small towns and villages in rural America.

Coinciding with the rise of specialization in medicine and the spread of intensive and coronary care units in the late 1960s, fewer physicians were choosing to enter general practice. Instead, increasing numbers of doctors were choosing to work in specialties such as cardiology, neurosurgery, and nephrology and were clustering near medical centers in cities and suburbs. Meanwhile, as the trend drew increasing numbers of physicians away from primary care, "report after report issued by the American Medical Association (AMA) and the Association of American Medical Colleges . . . decried the shortage of physicians in poor rural and urban areas."[10] At the same time, consumers across the nation were demanding accessible, affordable, and sensitive health care, while health care delivery costs were increasing at an annual rate of 10 percent to 14 percent.[11] Indeed, many considered the US health care system to be "too specialized, too centralized and inaccessible, too impersonal and too disease oriented."[12] The problem was that incentives in income, status, and lifestyle for physicians favored specialization.[13]

Concurrent with these trends, in 1965, federal funds made available under President Lyndon B. Johnson's "Great Society" ensured financial support for programs designed to reach the poor. Part of that funding, begun a year earlier, included the Nurse Training Act of 1964 (HB 10042), which authorized millions of dollars over five years for nursing school construction, special projects and planning grants, student loans and scholarships, and professional nurse traineeships. Its purpose was to strengthen and coordinate "existing programs aiding nurses' education with a major new nationwide effort to alleviate critical shortages of nurses required for the health care of all citizens."[14]

The funding came at a time when the nursing profession was struggling over two major issues: (1) educational preparation for entry-level practice, and (2) the purpose and focus of graduate nursing education. In 1965, the American Nurses' Association (ANA) had unilaterally declared the Bachelor of Science in Nursing (BSN) the "entry into practice" degree,[15] a decision that was "by no means universally accepted by the profession."[16] In fact, many nurse educators favored associate degree (two-year) and diploma school (three-year) preparation instead of the ANA's proposed four-year collegiate education. At the graduate level, nursing faculty were opening clinical nurse specialist programs in such areas as cardiac, neuro-surgical, and nephrology nursing. Professors of nursing were also interest-ed in identifying the nature of nursing and scope of practice, its theoreti-cal frameworks, and "the differentiation between 'caring' and 'curing.'"[17] So, when Ford and Silver introduced the idea of the pediatric nurse prac-titioner—a nurse who would diagnose and prescribe in addition to pro-moting well-child care—nurse faculty were concerned.[18]

## Controversy in Academia

For nearly a century, the nursing profession had been working to define its identity—separate from medicine. Now, faced with the concept of a nurse practitioner, "the great majority of America's nursing deans were outraged. . . . To [them], the concept meant that the nurses would become 'physician extenders,' and that the profession would lose ground in its struggle to escape subordination to medicine."[19] Tenured graduate faculty, "the power bloc in most schools,"[20] supported the emerging clinical nurse specialist (CNS) role instead. Introduced by Frances Reiter in 1943 in an effort to return expert nurses to direct patient care, the CNS role epito-mized clinical expertise in the profession. Many faculty wanted to reserve that title for nurses with a master's education.[21] Despite the opposition, other members of the faculty forged ahead with the establishment of NP programs (outside master's programs) within their schools. Based on the Colorado project, post-BSN certificate programs sprang up throughout the country. According to Ford:

> Although the initial goal . . . was to prepare nurses on the master's level for expert practice, teaching and clinical research, that intent was altered in order to accommodate the pressing societal demands for health care. Shortly thereafter, came an explosion of quickly gen-erated, short-term continuing education programs (some of which were devoid of academic standards) and products of variable quality. All of these programs used the name "practitioner." Hence, adult nurse practitioners, school nurse practitioners, family nurse practi-tioners and others came into being before the first pediatric nurse practitioner project was completely evaluated.[22]

In short, many programs awarded students an NP certificate after a few months of training. Students were not required to complete a master's degree in nursing (MSN), yet they would work in an expanded, "advanced" role after they received the certificate.[23]

Faculty concern over the focus of graduate education in nursing masked the underlying issue—the separation of the discipline of nursing from that of medicine. This issue manifested itself in the controversy over the fact that nurse practitioners made "medical" diagnoses and prescribed medications, blurring the boundaries between medicine and nursing. Professor and theorist Martha Rogers, RN, PhD, was one of the most outspoken opponents of the NP concept, arguing that the NP role undermined nursing's unique role in health care.[24]

While nursing professors addressed these issues—debating them in the literature, in national conferences, and in endless faculty meetings—professional groups and policy makers saw the possibilities of using NPs to solve the "access to care" problems in rural America.[25] Health policy groups, such as the National Advisory Commission on Health Manpower, issued statements in support of the NP concept.[26] All agreed that an ideal system would be staffed by "a mix of health care providers whose roles were different from the traditional roles of the 1960s."[27] Shortly thereafter, three innovations were introduced into the health care system: the nurse practitioner, "family medicine" as a new medical specialty, and the physician's assistant."[28]

If nurses in academe were upset about NPs, they were even more reactive to the role of the physician's assistant (PA) when Dr. Eugene Stead introduced it at Duke University in North Carolina in 1965. Senior nursing faculty at Duke refused to consider a nurse-practitioner program. In addition, the NLN refused to accredit an NP program. According to Stead: "The idea of having an NP program for medical surgical nursing at Duke, modeled after the PNP program established at Colorado, collapsed because the National League of Nursing (NLN) refused to accredit a program in which physicians would teach much of the curriculum.[29] Frustrated by the nursing community's refusal to collaborate to create this new medical-surgical nurse practitioner, the physicians who conceived of the idea concluded that the nurse leaders were "antagonistic to innovation and change" and initiated a physician's assistant (PA) program instead.[30] Physician's assistants (often experienced medical corpsmen who had just returned from Vietnam) would share the knowledge base formerly "owned" by medicine, but they would work under the license of the supervising physician.[31] Relationships between PAs and NPs, at least at the academic level, continued to be fraught with tension as more programs developed. By contrast, at the grassroots level, physician's assistants and nurse practitioners began to work together.

Practicing physicians accepted both the PA and the NP. In Lorraine Durran's case, the local physicians "welcomed her assignment" to the area, aware that she would improve health services to the Indians in Colorado.[32]

Educators might continue to argue over whether or not to prepare NPs in master's programs, and whether or not the NPs could diagnose and prescribe, but it was too late. Across the nation, in individual practices, nurse practitioners and physicians were already working together in what would be called "primary care" in the future.[33]

Furthermore, studies were already being done to evaluate PNPs' effectiveness. In 1967, one study determined that PNPs were highly competent in assessing and managing 75 percent of well and ill children in community health settings. In addition, PNPs increased the number of clients served in private pediatric practice by 33 percent.[34]

## An Idea Takes Hold

By the 1970s, Ford and Silver's idea took hold. It seemed logical to use the two major health care professions, medicine and nursing, together to expand primary care. People living in rural areas needed health care providers, and local physicians were interested. So was the federal government. In the early 1970s, Health, Education, and Welfare Secretary Elliot Richardson established the Committee to Study Extended Roles for Nurses and charged it with evaluating the feasibility of expanding nursing practice.[35]

The committee concluded that extending the scope of the nurse's role was essential to providing equal access to health care for all Americans. According to a 1971 editorial on the topic in the *American Journal of Nursing:* "The kind of health care Lillian Wald began preaching and practicing in 1893 is the kind the people of this country are still crying for. . . ."[36] The committee's report, published in November 1971, urged the establishment of innovative curricular designs for NP education in health science centers and increased financial support for nursing education.[37] It also urged national certification for nurse practitioners and developed a model nurse practice law that could be applied throughout the nation. In response, with mounting concern over the restrictive 1955 ANA definition of nursing practice, the ANA council suggested the following addendum to state nurse practice acts:

> A professional nurse may also perform such additional acts, under emergency or other special conditions, which may include special training, as are recognized by the medical and nursing professions as proper to be performed by a professional nurse under such condition, even though such acts might otherwise be considered diagnoses and prescription.[38]

Despite the cumbersome language, the addendum's meaning was clear: Intensive care nurses (including CCU nurses) could interpret electrocardiograms, defibrillate, start IVs, and give life-saving drugs according to standing orders. Nurse practitioners could diagnose and prescribe—as long as these acts were done under "special" conditions.

The Committee to Study Extended Roles for Nurses also called for further research related to cost-benefit analyses of the new role, as well as attitudinal surveys to assess its impact. The result was increased federal support for training programs for the preparation of several types of nurse practitioners, including family nurse practitioners (FNPs), adult nurse practitioners (ANPs), and emergency nurse practitioners (ENPs), among others.[39]

## Private Funding and Demonstration Projects

Funding these programs was another matter altogether, and much of that funding came from private foundations. One such, the Robert Wood Johnson (RWJ) Foundation, was aware of the resistance of the NLN and the nursing professors. Nonetheless, committed to supporting the NP movement, the Foundation initiated a series of regional demonstration projects focused on the training and deployment of nurse practitioners. Begun in the early 1970s, the programs were "intended to move [the NP-physician team] from an experimental, single-site stage [in Colorado] to patient care networks covering many sites."[40] The University of California, Davis; the Utah Valley Hospital, Provo; the Tuskegee Institute, Montgomery, Alabama; the University of Tennessee Medical Center, Memphis; and the Frontier Nursing Service in Hyden, Kentucky were among those funded. Their purpose was to implement broad-based community networks of primary care clinics using nurse practitioners.[41]

All of the sites had special characteristics that made them excellent choices for demonstration projects. The University of California–Davis was a "land-grant institution that embodied the tradition of community service" and had a medical school specifically to prepare physicians for rural practice; Utah Valley Hospital had already organized a network of rural clinics; and Tuskegee, "under the leadership of Dr. Cornelius Hopper, became the base for a three-county rural health system employing state of the art communications technology."[42] However, the Robert Wood Johnson Foundation couldn't have made a better choice for a model project than the Frontier Nursing Service. The FNS had a long history of meeting the health care needs of rural families in Appalachia using an established network of clinics. (See chapter 3.) Besides, the FNS was interested. According to the

RWJ Foundation: "With the advent of the nurse practitioner movement, the FNS decided that it would be advantageous for its staff and students to have dual training as family nurse practitioners."[43]

## The FNS Opens a Family Nurse-Practitioner Program

During the winter of 1969, the management consultant firm Booz, Allen, and Hamilton evaluated the "health manpower situation in Kentucky (particularly in the Eastern portion of the state)" as well as "the present and future" role of the Frontier Nursing Service.[44] After an extensive study, the firm concluded that (1) there was "a serious shortage of physicians and professional nurses in Kentucky, particularly in low income rural areas of the state"; (2) the FNS service had "demonstrated for nearly half a century the value of using a specially trained health worker to provide primary health care under the supervision of the physician"; and (3) the FNS had "proven its effectiveness in training nurse-midwives" for over 30 years.[45]

Based on their findings, the management consultants recommended that the "FNS Graduate School of Midwifery be 'expanded and modified . . . as part of a master's degree program in comprehensive family nursing . . . through university affiliation, preferably with the University of Kentucky' and that the FNS should establish a 'graduate program in comprehensive family nursing' and graduate 'about 25 family nurse practitioners per year.'"[46]

With financial backing from Robert Wood Johnson, the FNS family nurse-practitioner certificate program (FNP) opened in 1970. "The first class entered in June of that year, and the school changed its name to the 'Frontier School of Midwifery and Family Nursing (FSMFN)' to reflect its broadening educational role."[47] According to the school catalog, the "FNP would be a blending of nursing with selected medical and public health functions." The traditional nursing role would be expanded to include basic diagnostic, treatment and preventive skills so that FNPs would be "able to provide assistance to families, whether they be living in Appalachia, inner cities or developing countries. . . . "[48] With support from a three-year Primex Grant (1972–75), the program graduated over eighty students by 1974. By 1975 the FNS staff included "four physicians, 7 nurse midwives, 7 family nurse practitioners, 9 nurse-midwives/FNPs, 19 RNs and 5 LPNs. Of the 16 family nurse practitioners, nine were on the district clinic staff and seven were on the hospital outpatient clinic staff." Together they served a population base of 15,000 and had over 66,000 patient care encounters in one year.[49]

## The FNS and Prescriptive Medications

Guided by *Medical Directives* (formerly *Medical Routines*), as they had been in the past, the newly certified FNS nurse practitioners (along with the midwives and RNs) managed approximately 80 percent of the ambulatory care patients, "providing comparable patterns of care" to that of physicians.[50] They also dispensed, furnished, and quasi-"prescribed" medicines—this time under a new system for the "Distribution of Drugs."[51]

Since the inception of the FNS in the 1920s, the FNS pharmacy had supplied each district clinic with stock quantities of the drugs authorized by the *Medical Routines*. The nurse would pour, label, and dispense the medicines according to the standing orders (in legal terms, doing so was both "dispensing" and "furnishing drugs"). However, the procedure was getting especially complicated now, because the FNS pharmacist needed copies of the prescriptions that the nurses were writing. The nurses could not simply hand the patient a packet of pills or a bottle of medicine, as they had in the past. The system was cumbersome and the process time consuming. Besides, errors were occurring, and keeping an accurate inventory was difficult. According to one description:

> . . . In her clinic, the nurse would have as many as 1000 Potassium Penicillin G 250 mg tablets, 2000 Ferrous Sulfate [iron] tablets, several pints of Gantrisin pediatric suspension [antibiotic sulfa drug], and in some cases, one or more gallons of elixir of Benadryl [antihistamine for colds and allergies]. After examining a patient and making a diagnosis, she had to count tablets, put [them] in containers, and write out and label a prescription. . . . The nurses were spending too much time . . . on the simple procedures of counting, pouring and labeling prescriptions . . . and errors were being made—such as inadequate labels of prescriptions . . . like . . . 'shake well.' . . . And the pharmacy had a difficult time . . . keeping an inventory.[52]

To address these problems, the FNS pharmacist developed a new system for distributing medications. It consisted of "pre-typed prescriptions and prepackaged medications with proper labels attached."[53] The nurse in each district determined the number of prepackaged units she needed to stock her clinic. Except for "controlled drugs" (narcotics), which the nurse had to pick up herself, the prepackaged medicines were delivered to the clinics by couriers.[54]

Some procedures in the new system were just like those in the past. The nurse saw the patient, diagnosed the condition, and consulted the medical directives. In the new system, however, instead of pouring medicines out of large bottles into smaller ones and labeling the bottles, the FNP used the prepackaged drugs. According to the protocol, she pulled "the proper prescription and corresponding medications," dispensed the drugs, and returned a second copy of "the prescriptions to the pharmacy each week by courier rounds."[55] As one pharmacist described the procedure:

> Prescriptions themselves were pre-typed with blanks for certain pieces of information the nurse would complete before dispensing the medication. On the prescription there is the name of the drug, strength and quantity dispensed, directions to the patient, and the international disease code number. On the label are the directions, name and strength of drug, lot number and expiration date. The second prescription is the prescription [that is returned to us] after the nurse practitioner or midwife has dispensed the drug. . . . They must indicate the name of the patient, age, address, and circle the appropriate disease code number. . . . When the pharmacists and physicians review the prescription, they first check to see that the prescription is filled out accurately. They then determine the disease by looking at the disease code and check to see if the proper medications have been dispensed. For example, [on one prescription] the nurse has written for Gantrisin Pediatric suspension. The disease circle is 381. We look up 381 and find that the number represents acute otitis media [ear infection]. The patient being four ears old, the Medical Directives recommend Gantrisin, Penicillin and a decongestant. . . . We [then check] to see if the nurse has given the patient the other two drugs. . . . In this case, the Directives were followed and the physician "then" [sic] signs the prescriptions. Had there been a question, the nurse would have been asked to explain.

The new system was tidy. The NP saw the patient, diagnosed the condition, chose the appropriate drug from a list of possibilities, computed the dose, and wrote two prescriptions, one for the patient and one to be returned to the pharmacy. She then discussed with the mother the administration of the drug, the times it was to be given, the side effects that might occur, and any other special instructions. The supervising physician reviewed her decisions and signed the prescriptions "once a week."[56]

## Academia Comes Along

While some of these early programs (like the Frontier Nursing Service) were graduating students and implementing new protocols for practice, university faculty continued to debate whether or not the NP concept was a good idea

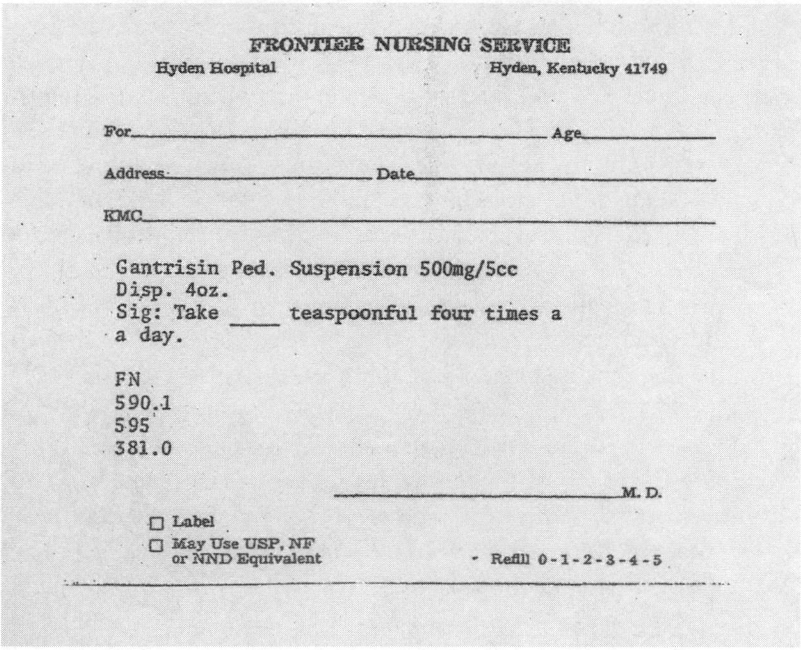

```
                    FRONTIER NURSING SERVICE
         Hyden Hospital                    Hyden, Kentucky 41749


    For_____  Age_____

    Address:_____ Date_____

    KMC_____


    Gantrisin Ped. Suspension 500mg/5cc
    Disp. 4oz.
    Sig: Take ____ teaspoonful four times a
    a day.

    FN
    590.1
    595
    381.0

                                     _____M. D.

       □ Label
       □ May Use USP, NF
         or NND Equivalent            • Refill 0 - 1 - 2 - 3 - 4 - 5
```

Figure 6.1: Sample prescription of gantrisin pediatric suspension. FNS, UK-SC

and whether or not NP education should take place in master's programs. In the late 1960s through the mid-1970s, most NP programs were the four-month, certificate-awarding variety.[57] Most were not housed in master's programs. However, there were a few exceptions. A "handful of leaders on graduate nursing faculties" envisioned primary care as an important new scholarly focus and supported the idea of incorporating the role into their master's degree programs. These faculty members, some of whom were deans, applied for funding from Robert Wood Johnson or supported other faculty in doing so. Among these deans and faculty members were Claire Fagin at the University of Pennsylvania; Ingeborg Mauksch at the University of Missouri at Columbia; Loretta Ford, who was now at Rochester University; and Rheba de Tornyay at the University of Washington. With their advice, the Foundation provided funds to Indiana University, Pace University, the University of Pennsylvania, the University of Rochester, Seton Hall University, and the University of Washington.[58]

In the late 1960s and through the 1970s, other schools applied for funding to the Division of Nursing, The United States Public Health Service (USPHS). The federal government was awarding grants under the Nurse Training Acts of 1965 and later of 1975 (P.L. 94–63). Title VIII, Section 822 of the 1975 Training Act specifically designated funds for NP education.[59]

The University of Pennsylvania was one institution that received funding from the RWJ Foundation. The program there, under the direction of Associate Professor Joan Lynaugh, graduated 136 students between 1978 and 1982.[60] Faculty at The University of Virginia (UVa) sought federal funding. Internist Dr. Reginia McCormick developed an adult NP program at UVa in 1970 (later administered by Dr. Robert Reed and Susan Lynch, RN). In 1972, Assistant Professor of Nursing Barbara Brodie and pediatrician Jake Lohr received Division of Nursing funding to open a PNP program within the nursing school's master's program. The University of Virginia later opened an emergency nurse-practitioner program, the first in the nation, directed by Denise Geolot, RN, MSN, and Richard Edlich, MD, director of emergency medical services at UVa.[61] All were supported by the Division of Nursing. By the end of 1978, the Division of Nursing was supporting eleven nurse-practitioner programs. An increasing number of these were master's programs—the majority of which were in the specialty areas of family and pediatric nursing.[62] Academia had come along after "ten years of intra-disciplinary argument."[63] In 1974, a group of faculty met in Chapel Hill, North Carolina, in the hopes of standardizing NP educational programs at the master's level.[64]

## Grassroots Collaboration and Negotiation

Individual physicians increasingly accepted NPs in their medical practices. Working together in offices and clinics, nurse practitioners and physicians established collegial relationships, negotiating with each other to construct work boundaries and define the terms of their collaborative practice. Nurse practitioners shared clinical decision-making skills with physicians, "collecting data through physical examination and history taking, ordering diagnostic laboratory tests and x-rays, formulating diagnoses and prescribing treatments"[65]—tasks that had defined the practice of medicine for centuries—or at least since the founding of the AMA.

According to historian Julie Fairman, "In the NP-MD dyad, negotiations centered on the NP's right to practice an essential part of traditional medicine: the process or skill set of clinical thinking . . . to perform a physical examination, elicit patient symptoms . . . create a diagnosis, formulate treatment options, prescribe treatment and make decisions about prognosis."[66] In these negotiations, NPs repeatedly explained "their role, education and experience, scope of practice, knowledge and skills."[67] The nurses (mostly young women) also had to maintain a "delicate balance between autonomy/control, paternalism, sexism, and supervision and

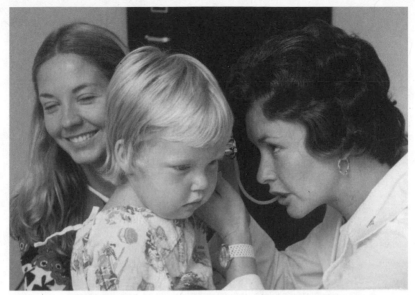

Figure 6.2: Barbara Dunn, PNP, examining child's ear, 1970s. CNHI

were continually challenged to insist on their bottom-line autonomy of the NP role."[68] Close proximity of the NP and physician was thought to be necessary, and "on-site" supervision was the norm (that is, if the practice setting was not in Appalachia or on a remote Indian reservation). According to early nurse practitioner Corene Johnson, "initially, we had to always have a physician on site. . . . I didn't resent that. Actually, I needed the backup."[69]

## Interprofessional Conflict over Prescriptive Authority

Although nurse practitioners and physicians were working together at the local level, conflict over the NP's scope of practice began to emerge at the organizational and state levels. One of the most contentious areas of inter-professional conflict involved prescriptive authority for nursing. Physicians did not want to give up control of the privilege of prescription. As a result, even when they were working together in close partnerships, both nurse practitioners and physicians danced around the issue of NPs writing prescriptions, just as they were doing in the Frontier Nursing Service. Nurse practitioners were, in fact, writing prescriptions, but both parties denied it by having physicians sign them—either all at once (as in the FNS protocol of having the doctor sign them at the end of the week) or one by one, in which case the physician hastily scribbled his signature on the prescription placed before him. When it was impossible to be "on-site" when the NP saw patients, or if it was simply more convenient to do so, the supervising physician sometimes handed the NP a pad of signed blank prescriptions for her use.[70] Much depended on whether or not the physician trusted the nurse's judgment. In other instances, physicians wrote and signed a specific prescription whenever NPs requested them to do so.[71] Except for the last, "all of these methods" were "of questionable legality."[72]

How prescriptions were handled depended on the availability of the physician, the negotiated boundaries of the individual physician-NP team, and the state in which practice occurred. In 1971, Idaho became the first state to recognize diagnosis and treatment as part of the scope of practice of specialty nurses but did not specifically recognize NPs or authorize them to write prescriptions.[73] According to law professor Barbara Safriet's later analysis, "as path-breaking as the statute was, it was still rather restrictive in that any acts of diagnosis and treatment had to be authorized by rules and regulations promulgated by the Idaho State Boards of Medicine and Nursing."[74] In other words, the practice of nursing by nurse practitioners would not be regulated by the Idaho State Board of Nursing, the usual body governing the practice of nursing. Instead, because NPs practiced in an expanded new role, the board of medicine joined with the board of nursing to regulate their practice. The situation was less than ideal, but it was a start. Getting state legislators to pass laws recognizing nurse practitioners would take time. In 1972, seven years after Ford and Silver opened the first formal NP program, only four state practice acts specifically mentioned the role. State by state, nurse practitioners would have to fight for the privilege of prescription. In 1975, North Carolina would be the first state to grant it.[75]

## Another Hurdle: Financial Reimbursement

Getting reimbursed by "third-party payers" for their services was another problem the nurse practitioners would have to face.[76] For years, NPs simply did not bill for their services but were paid instead by the physician (or institution) for whom they worked. There was no process that allowed the nurses to be reimbursed by insurance companies or other "third-party payers." The exception was the federal government, which could subsidize costs for the elderly and the poor, using the mechanism of Medicare and Medicaid, which were established in 1965. Later, the federal government subsidized care in rural and underserved areas. In 1976, the Indian Health Care Improvement Act was passed, with the goal of providing the highest possible health status to Indians. Comprehensive in scope, the Act authorized a number of programs that would serve as models for national health planning.[77] In 1977, Congress passed the Rural Health Clinicians Act (PL 95–210), allowing NPs (and physician assistants) who practiced in free-standing, physician-directed *rural* clinics located in areas with a shortage of health professionals to receive Medicare and Medicaid reimbursement for their services through payment to their physician employers.[78]

The Frontier Nursing Service took advantage of these funds, and other nursing leaders expressed their interest in doing so. Writing in her April 1979 report, Marlene Heffer, medical director of the Northern Arizona Indian Health Service, noted:

> The theme of the National Nursing Branch Chiefs meeting . . . was the "Rural Health Initiative." Nancy Lane, who helped to get the Rural Health Care Act passed through Congress, was the guest speaker. We discussed the desirability of developing some major initiatives for nursing and did propose three: home-health care, the use of nurse practitioners and discharge planning/coordination of services.[79]

Despite these advancements, the problem of reimbursement for NP services persisted. In fact, it got worse when the Reagan administration cut federal funding in the 1980s.

## Nurse Anesthetists, circa 1970s

While the nursing profession was preoccupied with the new nurse-practitioner role, nurse anesthetists continued to pursue their right to practice as part of an anesthesia team. In 1972, after years of negotiation, the American Association of Nurse Anesthetists (AANA) and the American Society of Anesthesiologists (ASA) issued the Joint Statement on Anesthesia Practice, promoting the concept of the anesthesia team. This statement coincided with the decision to place nurse anesthesia educational preparation in graduate programs for nursing. Nurse anesthesia met the requirements. It was an "expanded and advanced practice role" that required in-depth knowledge of pathophysiology, physical diagnosis, and advanced pharmacology, along with hundreds of hours of clinical practice. Moreover, the competencies that nurse anesthetists needed were much the same as those for the roles of nurse practitioner, clinical nurse specialist, and nurse-midwife, all of which would later be labeled "advanced practice" roles by the profession.[80] To achieve these, graduate training was deemed essential. In 1973, the University of Hawaii opened the first master's degree program for nurse anesthesia.

Because of the new requirements that nurse anesthetists have a master's degree in order to sit for national certification, many small certificate programs closed. Physician pressure, inadequate financial support, limited clinical facilities, and lack of accessible universities for affiliation also contributed to these closures.[81]

The economic implications of third-party payment would affect nurse anesthetists just as it did nurse practitioners. Beginning in 1977, the AANA led a long and complex effort to secure third-party reimbursement under Medicare so that nurse anesthetists could bill for their services.[82]

## Evaluating NP Practice

In order to get state legislators to vote for NP prescriptive authority, the nurses would have to document the safety and efficacy of their practice. In Colorado, Ford and Silver were already reporting on their results. In Philadelphia and Charlottesville, NP faculty were collecting data. In particular, nurse practitioners had to prove that their practice was safe. In a study reported in the *New England Journal of Medicine* in 1974, Repicky and colleagues reported "no difference between NPs and physicians in the 'adequacy' of their prescribing practices." In other words, the NPs' practice in prescribing medications was just as safe as that of the physicians.[83] Between 1970 and 1979, seventeen reports were published evaluating the NP role. These reports confirmed that NPs could be successfully integrated into various health care settings, provided "primary care services on a level with physicians," and were cost effective and acceptable to patients.[84] The studies reported on NP practice in a wide variety of settings and with different supervisory procedures. A study conducted by the NP faculty at the University of Virginia in 1978, for example, noted that the NPs rarely viewed x-rays, read EKGs, or prescribed medications independently.[85] However, another report noted that the medical needs of inner-city poor were "effectively and efficiently met by on-site nurse practitioners in telephone and television contact with supervising physicians."[86] All of the reports would be needed to convince state legislatures of the safety of NP practice. The most important one would come from the federal government in 1986.

## Changes in State Nurse Practice Acts

Using the reports of their safety and efficacy, nurse practitioners lobbied their states for changes to their practice acts to include the right to diagnose and prescribe. Because Idaho had been the first state to deal with the issue (albeit indirectly), and it had not given separate licensure to nurse practitioners, other states also did not. Instead, state legislatures instructed boards of medicine and nursing to draw up rules allowing nurse practitioners to practice.[87] Most determined that NPs should practice according to local protocols, much like those that the FNS nurses had been using for years. Others expanded their state's basic definition of all registered professional nurse practice, by either omitting or limiting the disclaimer in state practice acts against diagnosis and treatment by registered nurses. New York adopted this approach in 1972. The problem was that the states that did this sometimes did not mention nurse practitioners. Nurse practitioners would have to turn to the courts for clarification and support whenever their practice was questioned. A third approach to facilitating nurse practitioners' practice was to give more delegating powers to physicians through the state's medical practice act. Both Arizona and Colorado were among states using this tactic. Arizona also added an "additional acts" provision to give nurses permission to dispense drugs. According to that provision, the nurse was permitted to dispense

> prepackaged labeled drugs for a single medical episode under the direct order of a physician if (1) the nurse dispensing is employed or under contract with a county health officer, and (2) the dispensing is in rural areas of exceptional medical needs as defined by the board of medical examiners.[88]

Covered by law, a physician in Arizona could delegate responsibilities to an Indian Health Service nurse practitioner, and a pediatrician in Colorado could delegate specific medical acts to one of the newly employed pediatric nurse practitioners. The process worked. However, the NP's practice occurred under the physician's license instead of under that of the NP. And Arizona law's specific comments made the practice act more opaque. In striving for clarity, the legislators created ambiguity: what was a "single medical episode"? And did standing orders qualify as direct orders? These comments were actually undermining the intent of the law (i.e., recognizing the nurse practitioner's expanded role and permitting a nurse to act in this role only when there was no one else to perform it, for example, in areas of exceptional need).[89] The situation would become more complicated in 1984, when the American Medical Association House of Delegates passed a resolution to combat "any attempt at empowering non-physicians to become unsupervised primary care providers and be directly reimbursed."[90]

# CHAPTER 7

# Prescriptive Authority for Advanced Practice Nurses, 1980–2000

Subject: HB818 passed to third reading
Date: Tue, 8 Feb 2000 10:42:28–0500
From: [name] <email address>xyz.org
To: <Undisclosed Recipients@zeus.i-c.net>

Today, the House of Delegates [Virginia] passed HB-818, broadened prescriptive authority, from the second to the third reading on a voice vote. There were no amendments. We have no way of knowing how many of the 100 Delegates voted for HB-818. We have heard from a number of Delegates who are voting against the bill that we don't need their votes to get the bill passed. While none of us is taking anything for granted, we are cautiously optimistic about the House.

The next event: On Tuesday, we expect the bill will be voted on final passage from the House. That will be a recorded vote that we will distribute so you can see how your Delegate voted on HB-818.

There is some small chance that the bill could "go by for the day," or not be voted until later in the week. We will keep you posted.

Prior to today's vote, the Medical Society of Virginia had told us that they would have two amendments to HB-818 proposed on the floor today. One was to broaden prescriptive authority to include only Schedule V and VI drugs. The other was to specify additional education that would be necessary for NPs with broadened prescriptive authority. One of the arguments used by physicians against any expansion of NP scope of practice is that if NPs want to be doctors (i.e., prescribe), they should go to medical school. Therefore, we speculated that the additional educational requirement would be graduation from an accredited medical school, which the Medical Society denied.

HB-818 was heard immediately following a protracted debate on a patient's right to sue their Health Maintenance Organization (HMO), which by the way passed . . . The Delegates clearly were tired of sitting, and many got up and walked around. Apparently, no one had the appetite for prolonged debate on HB818, and the Medical Society's amendments never were proposed.

Here is an abbreviated version of the debate on this bill. Please keep in mind that accuracy is not always the hallmark of good debate on the floor. . . . [1]

In February 2000, e-mails about prescriptive authority for NPs were flying, most informing nurse practitioners of the latest news from the state capitol, where some NP representatives were closely following what was occurring on the House floor. Clearly, nurse practitioners across the Commonwealth of Virginia wanted their delegates to the House of Representatives to vote for a bill expanding NPs' prescriptive privileges. For years, nurse practitioners had been restricted from prescribing certain categories of drugs they needed to prescribe if they were to provide comprehensive care. In fact, NPs in thirty-four other states had broader prescriptive authority than did NPs in Virginia.

Since the implementation of the Controlled Substance Act of 1970, federal law categorized prescription drugs into two types: (1) legend drugs (like antibiotics—medicines that could be dispensed only by prescription, but which were not narcotics), and (2) narcotics or controlled substances listed on five schedules. Schedule I substances included illegal drugs like heroin; Schedule II were "drugs with significant addictive potential,"[2] like morphine, fentanyl, and oxycodone (commonly known as Percodan); Schedule III were drugs that had "some potential for abuse," including Tylenol with codeine, and opium combinations (Paregoric); Schedule IV drugs had "low potential for abuse but could lead to physical or psychological dependence,"[3] like alprazolam (Xanax), diazepam (Valium) and lorazepam (Ativan); Schedule V drugs included "drugs determined to have low abuse potential but designated for regulation by individual states and localities" because they contained limited quantities of certain narcotics.[4] These drugs included antidiarrheal compounds and cough medicines with codeine.

By 2000 non-narcotic *legend* drugs (like amoxicillin and other antibiotics) had become known as Schedule VI drugs. Schedule VI drugs also included over-the-counter medicines like ibuprofen (Advil).[5] The Virginia Medical Society's proposed amendment (that did not actually get to the floor) was to add only "Schedule V and VI" drugs, allowing NPs to prescribe such medicines as cough medicine with codeine (Schedule V), as well as antibiotics and drugs widely available to the public for self-administration—like aspirin, Vaseline, zinc oxide ointment, milk of magnesia, hydrogen peroxide, castor oil, Vicks VapoRub, and so on (Schedule VI). With the exception of antibiotics, the latter included drugs nurses had been dispensing and furnishing for over a century (see chapter 1).[6]

Nurse practitioners in Virginia were not pleased with the Medical Society's proposed amendment. Some, including acute care nurse practitioners (ACNPs), were working in hospital settings caring for acutely ill patients and needed to order narcotic drugs like fentanyl to relieve pain or drugs like Ativan to control seizures. Others were following patients in subspecialty clinics in cardiology, neurology, and oncology. Their patients needed a wide variety of medicines ranging from those in Schedule II to those in Schedule VI. For example, a cardiac patient often needed nitroglycerin tablets (Schedule VI) but could also require a Schedule II drug like morphine if he had an episode of severe chest pain. For nurse practitioners working in primary care settings, the right to prescribe a wide range of drugs was also important in order for them to administer comprehensive care in a timely manner. For example, patients sometimes needed Schedule III drugs like Tylenol with codeine for pain that was unresponsive to over-the-counter analgesics. Other patients with protracted coughs might need a cough medicine containing codeine. As more primary care providers were treating patients with psychological disorders, these NPs might also need to prescribe any of a wide variety of Schedule IV drugs (e.g., Xanax or Ativan).

The NPs in Virginia were asking for the privilege to prescribe all schedules of drugs, limited only by their supervising physician. In the nurses' proposal, the nurse practitioner would be permitted to prescribe only what her supervising physician agreed was "appropriate based on the kind of practice, the NP's experience and education, and the level of trust" the physician had in the NP.[7] In addition, as one nurse noted, "The Board of

Medicine and the Board of Nursing would jointly decide, in regulations, what additional education would be necessary for nurse practitioners with broadened prescriptive authority."[8] Nurse practitioners in Virginia were determined to get HB818 passed. They went so far as to meet with Emily Couric, the state senator for the 25th district, in her Charlottesville office the week before the Senate debate to discuss "the potential benefits such legislation would have for increasing access to health care services, particularly in rural and underserved areas."[9] Following the meeting, Senator Couric wrote to the NPs, assuring them that she would keep their "comments in mind" during the proposed debate.[10]

## Acknowledging and Authorizing Prescribing Practices

Since 1965, when the first PNPs began to practice, nurse practitioners had been striving for the legal authority to prescribe. The issue, of course, was not whether NPs *could* and *did* prescribe, but rather, whether states would "*acknowledge* and *authorize* their prescribing practices."[11] Except for Idaho, which was the first state to recognize diagnosis and treatment as part of the scope of practice of specialty nurses in 1971, and North Carolina, which explicitly authorized nurse practitioners to prescribe drugs in 1975,[12] state legislatures had been slow to respond.

Convincing state legislatures to pass laws and reimbursement policies that would support NP practice was not easy. The major issue was, as usual, control of medical practice and the degree of independence a nurse practitioner should be allowed. Generally, state medical practice acts broadly defined the physician's scope of practice to include curing, diagnosing, treating, and prescribing.[13] It was hard for the nurses not to be accused of practicing medicine if they did any of these activities. The issue could not simply be ignored. Nurse practitioners were already de facto prescribing, and physicians could accuse them of "practicing medicine without a license." As was true in the 1920s and 1930s, if the state laws regulating nursing practice did not specifically grant nurses the rights to diagnose and prescribe, nurses and physicians would have to turn to the courts for a decision whenever nursing practice was questioned.

### *Sermchief v. Gonzales*

As had been true in previous decades, in 1980 the Missouri Courts would be asked to decide on a question of nursing practice. That year, the Missouri State Board of Medicine charged two nurse practitioners working in a women's health clinic of practicing medicine without a license. In the course of their work at the clinic, the NPs, Ms. Solari and Ms. Burgess, had been taking health histories, doing breast and pelvic examinations, ordering laboratory tests, providing information to patients about contraception, and "dispensing certain designated medications . . . pursuant to written standing orders and protocols signed by physicians."[14]

The court ruled against the nurses,[15] finding them guilty of practicing medicine without a license. Its decision was based on the statute for the practice of medicine in Missouri in 1980, which included the following section:

> It shall be unlawful for any person not now a registered physician within the meaning of the law to practice medicine or surgery in any of its departments, or to profess to cure and attempt to treat the sick and others afflicted with bodily or mental infirmities, or engage in the practice of midwifery in this state, except as herein provided.[16]

The court had also used the statute on nursing practice in Missouri on which to base its decision. That statute included the following definition of professional nursing:

> "Professional nursing" is the performance for compensation of any act which requires substantial specialized education, judgment and skill based on knowledge and application of principles derived from the biological, physical, social and nursing sciences, including, but not limited to: (a) Responsibility for the teaching of health care . . . (b) Assessment, nursing diagnosis, nursing care and counsel of persons who are ill, injured or experiencing alterations in normal health processes; (c) The administration of medications and treatments as prescribed by a person licensed in this state to prescribe such medications and treatments; (d) The coordination and assistance in the delivery of a plan of care . . . ; or (e) The teaching and supervision of other persons in the performance of any of the foregoing.[17]

Following their loss in the lower court, the nurses appealed to the Missouri Supreme Court. They were supported by *amicus curiae* briefs "resembling a letter-writing campaign directed at a legislative body."[18] Summarizing the content of those briefs in the final report, the judges wrote: "It suffices to say that those briefs detailed the historical development of the nursing profession and the nurses' expanding role in the delivery of health services, the reality of which both the Court and the public notice. Many expressed their opinions as to how we should construe our

Missouri statues, a matter which we are obligated to do in accordance with long established rules of statutory construction."[19]

Clearly irritated by the sheer volume of *amicus curiae* briefs, the Missouri Supreme Court judges went on to note a new procedure and rules for submitting them, then returned to a discussion of the issue at hand:

> The facts are simple . . . the appellant nurses Solari and Burgess are duly licensed professional nurses in Missouri . . . both have had postgraduate training in the field of obstetrics and gynecology . . . Appellant physicians . . . are duly licensed. . . . The ultimate issues for determination [are]: (A) does the conduct of plaintiff nurses Solari and Burgess constitute Professional Nursing as defined in #335.016.8 [the nurse practice act] . . . and (B) If the court finds and concludes that any act of the plaintiffs does not constitute "professional nursing" . . . the Court must determine if #334.010 [the medical practice act] is unconstitutionally vague. . . .

> The parties on both sides request that in construing these statutes we define and draw that thin and elusive line that separates the practice of medicine and the practice of nursing in modern day delivery of health services. . . . In our opinion [that] would result in an avalanche of both medicine and nursing malpractice suits alleging infringement of that line and would hinder . . . the delivery of health services to the public.[20]

In the end, the court decided in favor of the nurses, reasoning:

> Fundamentally, we seek to ascertain the intent of the lawmakers and to give effect to that intent. . . . The legislature substantially revised the law affecting the nursing profession with enactment of the Nursing Practice Act of 1975. Perhaps the most significant feature of the Act was the redefinition of the term "professional nursing," which appears in #335.016.8. Even a facile reading of that section reveals a manifest legislative desire to expand the scope of authorized nursing practices. Every witness at trial testified that the new definition of professional nursing is a broader definition than that in the former statute. . . . Most apparent is the elimination of the requirement that a physician directly supervise nursing functions. Equally significant is the legislature's formulation of an open-ended definition of professional nursing. . . . The 1975 Act not only describes a much broader spectrum of nursing functions [than earlier legislation], it qualifies

this description with the phrase "including, but not limited to." We believe this phrase evidences an intent to avoid statutory constraints on the evolution of new functions for nurses delivering health services. Under #335.016.8, a nurse may . . . assume responsibilities heretofore not considered to be within the field of professional nursing so long as those responsibilities are consistent with her or his "specialized education, judgment and skill based on knowledge and application of principles derived from the biological, physical, social and nursing sciences."[21]

The Missouri Supreme Court decision would set precedent for nursing practice for the remainder of the century. New state nurse practice acts used very general wording to allow for expansion in nurses' roles and functions over time. They also defined professional nursing to include the acts of diagnosis and treatment—a significant ruling for nurse practitioners.

## "Nursing Diagnosis" and Nurse Practice Acts

The general wording and the expanded functions listed in the 1975 Missouri Nurse Practice Act were critical to the judges' decision. One of the new terms, "nursing diagnosis," was particularly important, although it would have been equally effective had the statute used the terms "diagnosis" or "medical diagnosis," as other states would later do. Nevertheless, in 1975 the Missouri legislators drafting the nurse practice act used the term that was just being developed. In fact, the Missouri definition was one of the first to include it, as the Nursing Diagnosis movement was in its infancy. In 1973, nurse leaders Kristine Gebbie and Mary Ann Lavin had convened the First Task Force to Name and Classify Nursing Diagnoses and appointed Marjory Gordon, PhD, RN, as chairperson. In 1974, the First Conference Proceedings, edited by Gebbie and Lavin, were published.[22]

Nursing was still trying to carve out its niche but differentiate its practice from the medical model, and many nurses were determined to draw that "thin and elusive line" (as it was described by the Missouri Supreme Court) between the professions. Differentiating nursing from medical diagnoses was one step toward drawing that line, and, although it would lead to controversy within the profession, in this case, the incorporation of the particular term had been critical to the nurses' success.

## State Nurse Practice Acts and NP Practice: 1980s

Although states soon incorporated the acts of diagnosis and treatment into their laws regulating nursing practice, a large majority continued to avoid granting nurses independent prescriptive authority. By 1983, only Oregon and Washington granted NPs statutory independent prescriptive authority. Other states granting prescriptive authority to nurse practitioners did so with the provision that the nurse practitioner be directly supervised by a licensed physician. Particularly in the 1980s, when federal funding for health care services decreased under the Reagan administration, it was—as Elizabeth Hadley noted—in the "economic best interest" of physicians to confine NPs to a "largely complementary role in the provision of health services."[23]

By 1984, approximately 20,000 NPs were employed, for the most part in outpatient clinics, health maintenance organizations (HMOs), health departments, community health centers, rural clinics, schools, occupational health clinics, and private offices.[24] The problem was that many worked under various titles, including "nurse clinician," "advanced clinical nurse," and "nurse practitioner." Moreover, all of these titles had different meanings, differing descriptions of educational requirements, and different performance expectations.[25] The issue plagued the profession and was hotly debated in the nursing literature. As Yale law professor Barbara Safriet later noted, the "multiplicity of roles and titles for advanced practice nurses (APNs)" resembled "the rubble of the Tower of Babel." According to Safriet, "Even the most sophisticated health care consumer or policymaker" could be "easily confused."[26] Nursing as a profession had to clarify its titles and its educational requirements for advanced practice before legislators could be expected to write meaningful laws regulating its practice.[27]

Before Safriet's commentary, nurses themselves realized the confusion that the plethora of new titles was causing. In 1984, Joy Calkin, associate professor at the University of Wisconsin–Madison, proposed a model for advanced nursing practice, specifically identifying clinical nurse specialists and nurse practitioners with master's degrees as advanced practice nurses, or APNs.[28] Other practitioners, including nurse anesthetists and nurse-midwives with graduate education, would soon share the title. By definition, advanced practice nurses were educated at the master's level, worked in direct clinical practice, were expert coaches, provided consultation, used research to determine practice, provided clinical and professional leadership, collaborated with other professionals, and used ethical decision making.[29] For those who would be certified as nurse practitioners, part of their education included classes in advanced health assessment and physical diagnosis, as well as advanced pharmacology. In addition, they had hundreds of hours of clinical application.

## Opposition from the American Medical Association

While the nursing profession was striving for clarity in role definitions and titles, graduating nurse practitioners, nurse anesthetists, and nurse-midwives with master's degrees and watching them become employed in various settings, the American Medical Association was planning to "combat" new legislation that authorized "medical acts by unlicensed individuals."[30] In fact, in 1984 the AMA House of Delegates passed a resolution to "oppose any attempt at empowering non-physicians to become unsupervised primary care providers and be directly reimbursed."[31] According to that resolution:

> The AMA (1) opposes the enactment of new legislation which would authorize the independent practice of medicine by individuals who are not licensed to practice medicine and surgery in all of its branches; and (2) supports the enactment of amendments to restrict current statutes which authorize the independent practice of medicine by individuals who are not licensed to practice medicine and surgery in all of its branches.[32]

To block new legislation to this effect, the AMA would have to lobby state legislators. By tradition, state governments controlled medical and nursing practice.[33] Regulations varied according to each state. Some states allowed nurse practitioners to practice independently, whereas others restricted them to practice only under physician supervision.[34] Constraints included "requirements for written agreements and written protocols, a limited selection of drugs listed in an official formulary" that was itself "limited to Schedule VI drugs and devices, and supervision by a physician."[35]

For the remaining years of the twentieth century, both individual physicians and medical associations *did* lobby against "any legislative efforts to acknowledge prescriptive authority as part of the advanced practice nurses' scope of practice."[36] To make it easier to do so, in April 1992 the AMA adopted model legislation on the "Regulation of Prescription-Writing Authority of Nurse Practitioners," defining prescribing as a medical act.[37]

## Nursing Publications and Cost-Effective Care

Members of the nursing profession decided to argue for the safety and efficacy of NP practice using scientifically based research data. Since the 1950s, as increasing numbers of nurse faculty were educated at the PhD level, they had been emphasizing clinical research, conducting studies, and publishing their results. By the 1970s, among other things, they were conducting studies on NPs' practice. By 1980, nurse researchers studying nurse practitioners' effectiveness had documented that their care was comparable to that of physicians.[38] Throughout the 1980s, nurses published about the unique aspects of NP practice that distinguished it from medical practice, particularly about the cost-effectiveness of care provided by the nurses.[39]

Cost containment in health care characterized the 1980s, producing legislative and economic changes that affected the entire health care delivery system. Of particular significance was the establishment in 1983 of a prospective payment system using diagnosis-related groups (DRGs) for hospitalized Medicare recipients. In an effort to control rising hospital costs, this payment system shifted reimbursement from "payment for services provided" to "payment by case" (capitation). As a result, hospital administrators pressured nurses and physicians to decrease the length of time patients remained in the hospital. The hospital would be reimbursed for the "disease condition," based on standardized estimates of what the treatment should cost, rather than for the amount of time it took for the patient to be ready for discharge. Each day the patient stayed in the hospital cut the hospital's profit margin.

In the mid-1980s, the need to provide cost-effective, quality care to American citizens prompted the US Senate Committee on Appropriations to request a report from the Office of Technology and Assessment (OTA) on the contributions of nurse practitioners, certified nurse-midwives, and physician's assistants in meeting the nation's health care needs. The report, released in 1986 and entitled "Nurse Practitioners, Physician Assistants and Certified Nurse Midwives" (later referred to as the OTA Report), was based on an analysis of numerous studies that assessed quality of care, as well as patient satisfaction and physician acceptance. It concluded that "within their areas of competence NPs . . . and CNMs [certified nurse-midwives] provide care whose quality is equivalent to that of care provided by physicians."[40] Unfortunately, the OTA Report only compared nursing care to medical care and did not address the "value-added" components of advanced nursing practice—particularly the holistic perspective, health promotion, and patient education.[41]

The OTA Report also found that the cost of care provided by nurse practitioners (per care episode) was 20 percent less than traditional physician-provided care for the same patient population. The problem was that nurse practitioners could not be reimbursed by third-party payers. There was another problem: while the OTA was conducting its study, the American Medical Association was taking a stance against nonphysician care providers. Primary care was becoming a medical specialty.[42]

## Nurse Anesthetists, circa 1980s

While the profession as a whole focused on nurse practitioners, the specialty of nurse anesthesia continued to develop. By 1980 there were four master's programs in nurse anesthesia in the United States.[43] Despite this progress on the educational front, interprofessional conflicts with medicine continued. Although the earlier litigation, *Frank et al. v. South*[44] and *Chalmers-Frances v. Nelson*,[45] provided the critical legal basis of nurse anesthesia practice, tension between medicine and nurse anesthetists continued, particularly in relation to malpractice policies, antitrust, and restraint of trade issues. In 1986, *Oltz v. St. Peter's Community Hospital* established that certified registered nurse anesthetists (CRNAs) could sue for anticompetitive damages when anesthesiologists conspired to restrict the CRNAs' practice privileges. A second case, *Bhan v. NME Hospitals, Inc.*,[46] established the CRNAs' right to be awarded damages when hospital administrators made exclusive contracts with physician anesthesiologists—contracts that barred CRNAs from practicing there. As evidenced in all these cases, nurse anesthetists were winning the legal battles and overcoming barriers to their practice.

Like nurse practitioners during the 1980s, nurse anesthetists also had to overcome barriers to be reimbursed for their services by third-party payers. The chief problem was that nurse anesthetists could not bill for their services, and hospital administrators had to consider them as a cost center rather than as a revenue-generating service, creating reimbursement disincentives for their employment.[47]

## 1990s: The Challenges of Managed Care

The changing marketplace of the 1990s, with its focus on health care reform, created new challenges for nurse practitioners. Now they had to struggle not only with restrictive, outdated state laws on prescriptive authority, but also with "non-governmental, market-based impediments" to their practices.[48] Writing in *The Yale Journal on Regulation* in 1992, Barbara J. Safriet urged immediate legislative reform to reduce the restrictions on advance practice nurses, particularly those constraining the work of nurse practitioners and certified nurse-midwives.[49] According to Safriet:

> Although our ailing health care system presents an endless array of symptoms, the diagnosis is relatively straightforward: too few people can get good care when they need it and at a price they can afford. Any proposed cure should therefore include, at a minimum, steps to

eliminate . . . those things that impede the efficient and effective provision of health care. . . . Chief among these are conflicting and
restrictive state provisions governing the scope of practice and prescriptive authority of Nurse Practitioners and Certified Nurse
Midwives (CNMs), as well as the fragmented and parsimonious state
and federal standards for their reimbursement. As a result of these
provisions, NPs and CNMs are severely hampered—or disabled altogether—in their efforts to fulfill their fully proven potential to
enhance our nation's health.[50]

One of those restrictions had to do with controlled substances.

## The Controlled Substances Act, 1991–92

Federal legislation regulating narcotics in the Controlled Substances Act
(revised in 1991 and 1992), would play a major role in the nurse practitioner's attempt to obtain prescriptive authority during the 1990s. As nurse
practitioners began to gain prescriptive authority for controlled substances
in the different states, they required a parallel authority granted by the
Federal Drug Enforcement Agency (DEA). In 1991, the DEA first
responded to this situation by proposing registration for "affiliated practitioners" (56FR 4181). This proposal called for those nurse practitioners
who had prescriptive authority pursuant to a practice protocol or collaborative practice agreement to be assigned a registration number for controlled substances tied to the numbers of physicians with whom they
worked. The proposal was criticized for restricting access to health care and
its implications for legal liability. Because of these problems, it was revoked
early in 1992. Later, in July of that year, the DEA amended its regulations
by adding a category of "mid-level providers" (MLP), to include advanced
practice nurses, who would be issued *individual* provider DEA numbers so
long as they were granted prescriptive authority by the state in which they
practiced. The mid-level provider's number would begin with an "M." The
provision took effect in 1993, significantly expanding the NPs' ability to
prescribe.

By 1994, over 50,000 nurse practitioners were practicing as primary
care providers and had negotiated some form of prescriptive authority in
forty-six states. Twenty-five states had legislation authorizing private and
commercial insurers to reimburse them for their services, twenty-one states
and the District of Columbia permitted them to write prescriptions for
drugs, and fifteen of these gave independent prescribing authority for controlled substances.[51] Alaska and Oregon gave full prescriptive powers to

advanced practice nurses permitting them to practice independently of physician control. Most other states, including New York, limited their autonomy by requiring nurse practitioners to practice in collaboration with a licensed physician.[52] According to the New York state practice act:

> The practice of registered professional nursing by a nurse practition-er, certified under section six thousand nine hundred ten of this arti-cle, may include the diagnosis of illness and physical conditions and the performance of therapeutic and corrective measures within a spe-cialty area of practice, in collaboration with a licensed physician qualified to collaborate in the specialty involved, provided such serv-ices are preformed in accordance with a written practice agreement and written practice protocols. . . . [53]

"Specialty areas of practice" would soon expand from primary care to include numerous specialties such as neurology, neurosurgery, cardiology, nephrology, and intensive care, as the idea of using nurse practitioners in tertiary care centers was on the horizon.


## Acute Care Nurse Practitioners

As health care became increasingly based on technology, and as patients progressed rapidly from intensive care units to "step-down" units to home in an attempt to decrease their length of stay, hospital care lacked conti-nuity and coordination. In fact, patients were cared for by numerous teams of doctors and nurses. One particular nurse did not follow the patient from admission to discharge in order to have a complete picture of what the patient had been through during hospitalization and what the plan was for care afterwards. Doctors were rushed and often busy in sur-gery or busy following other patients in clinics. Patient care was becoming increasingly fragmented as specialists came and went, seeing the patient for only one particular problem.

A few nurse educators responded quickly to the problem, creating a role that was to provide quality patient care and care coordination.[54] Their solution was to put nurse practitioners inside hospitals. University of Pennsylvania Professor Anne Keane and Theresa Richmond, RN, MSN, were among the first to document the new "Tertiary Nurse Practitioner" (TNP) role, writing:

> The TNP is an advanced practice nurse educated at the master's level with both a theoretical and experiential focus on complex patients

with specialized health needs. . . . There is precedent for the NP in tertiary care. For example, neonatal nurse practitioners are central to the provision of care in many intensive care nurseries. . . . It is our belief that the TNP can provide clinically expert specialized care in a holistic manner in a system that is often typified by fragmentation, lack of communication among medical specialists and a loss of recognition of the patient and patient's needs as central to the care delivered.[55]

It was a logical next step. Nurse practitioners were already working in the outpatient setting and in neonatal intensive care clinics with premature newborns, and their care had been proven to be effective.[56] Now, nurse practitioners who wanted to work with adult patients inside the hospital could become "TNPs," a title that was quickly changed to "Acute Care Nurse Practitioners," or ACNPs. These nurses were usually experienced in caring for patients in various medical specialties, like cardiology, nephrology, neurology, and oncology. Some had been clinical nurse specialists for years and now wanted to have the skills and knowledge necessary to follow patients in specialty clinics. They needed to have the skills to take health histories and prescribe medications in addition to doing the patient education and counseling they were already doing. Those skills could be acquired in nurse-practitioner programs.

Nurse faculty responded by creating acute care nurse practitioner tracks within their master's programs. Between 1992 and 1995, numerous ACNP programs opened. In 1995, the American Nurses Credentialing Center (ANCC) administered the first ACNP certification examination.[57] By the late 1990s, acute care nurse practitioners were employed in multiple specialties, including, among others, cardiology, cardiovascular surgery, neurosurgery, emergency/trauma, oncology, internal medicine, and radiology services.[58] Meanwhile, the idea of requisite master's preparation for nurse anesthetists was also becoming a reality.

## Nurse Anesthetists in the 1990s

As the decade opened, there were seventeen master's programs in nurse anesthesia; by 1999, there were eighty-two.[59] As of 1998, all accredited programs in nurse anesthesia were required to be at the master's level; however, they were not uniformly located within schools of nursing. Rather, they were housed in a variety of disciplines, including schools of nursing, medicine, allied health, and basic science. As it had been throughout the century, nurse anesthetist programs continued to be regarded by the profession as "on the fringe." Toward the turn of the twenty-first century, however, CRNA programs were increasingly becoming incorporated into graduate nursing programs.

## Conflict and Negotiations Continue

During the 1990s, conflict with the medical profession and negotiations with state legislatures continued. In 1994, Dr. Jerome Kassirer, writing in the *New England Journal of Medicine,* questioned the role of nurse practitioners in primary care. He particularly discredited the published data on the NPs' competency and effectiveness, and he accused the OTA Report of "serious flaws, including a lack of appropriate controls, heterogeneity of practice settings, small sample of nurse practitioner subjects and patients, lack of random assignment of patients, failure to account for differences in the severity of illnesses and a paucity of outcome events."[60] Kassirer also noted that he was not "the first to point out these shortcomings," as they were "described in the OTA report and by nurse researchers themselves" in their call for better-designed studies in the future. Kassirer did concede that NPs effectively managed "a large number of common problems" like sore throats, "with and without physician supervision." Kassirer argued that he was not concerned with "considerations of turf"; rather, he was concerned with the fact that the nurse practitioners had considerably less training, and primary care was becoming more complicated. He argued that there were increasingly sophisticated diagnostic tests that needed a high level of education to interpret. Kassirer concluded with a statement of caution that the safety and efficacy of advanced practice nurse's care needed to be established before "further expanding an independent role for nurse practitioners."[61]

Dr. Kassirer had a point. With the knowledge explosion in the fields, both medicine and nursing were becoming increasingly complex. New drugs were being added to the formularies on a daily basis, and many practitioners, overwhelmed with information, were turning to the use of hand-held "Palm Pilots" or personal digital assistants (PDAs) to keep up with the new information.[62] Furthermore, Kassirer was justified in his argument for careful analysis of nurse practitioner practice through randomized, controlled clinical trials (RCTs) with larger sample sizes and homogeneity of practice settings and patient populations. RCTs are, of course, the "gold standard" for research studies and nurse researchers would agree that studies should be ongoing.

What Dr. Kassirer did not mention was that nurse practitioners are professionals who can be trusted to know the limits of their areas of competence and determine when they need physician consultation. As professionals, they could also be trusted to attend pharmacology seminars and continuing education conferences on new diagnostic tests and new therapies, and/or read the literature in their particular fields in order to ensure that they had the knowledge they needed to provide safe care—just as physicians are trusted to do.[63] Enhancing that legitimacy, state boards of nursing, or in some cases joint boards of nursing and medicine, were establishing criteria for nurse-practitioner licensure, and certification boards were determining who could sit for examination.

## Necessary Knowledge for Safe Care

Necessary knowledge for safe practice was indeed being mandated for the increasing numbers of NPs entering practice.[64] By 1994, 384 NP tracks were incorporated in master's programs throughout the United States. By 1998, that number was 769.[65] Most used the National Organization of Nurse Practitioner Faculty (NONPF) guidelines in determining curriculum[66]—guidelines that required nurse practitioners to have courses in advanced pathophysiology, physical assessment, and pharmacology and a minimum of five hundred hours of supervised clinical practice. As of the end of 1997, the ANA required that applicants who wanted to sit for advanced practice certification examinations have a minimum of master's level preparation. The reality was that many had post-master's educational preparation. Some had PhDs or other doctoral degrees (e.g., DNSc, ND). The nursing profession itself was cognizant of the fact that these practitioners would be expected to perform at an advanced level, and wanted that care to be safe.

## Realities of Practice

Nurse practitioners wrote fifteen million prescriptions in 1998, an increase of 66 percent over 1997, according to the pharmaceutical consulting firm Scott-Levin. Although the public debate over prescriptive authority was framed in terms of quality of care, economics was the subtext.[67] The market forces represented more significant barriers than regulatory ones. As law professor Barbara Safriet would note in 1998:

> No longer is governmental prohibition or restriction the only—or
> even the principal problem. Now an increase in the competitive chaos
> of the marketplace has thrown APNs into unfamiliar territory in

which private contracting, market-share, and capital requirements may pose potentially serious obstacles. From closed panels to physician-dominated contracting arrangements with integrated delivery systems, APNs and other "non-physician providers" face new non-governmental, market-based impediments to their practices.[68]

Nurse practitioners had been slowly making progress in removing legal barriers to practice. At the turn of the twenty-first century, many states were recognizing nurse practitioner practice and expanding the scope of prescriptive authority for advanced practice nurses. The Commonwealth of Virginia provides one example of what was occurring nationwide.

## The Virginia Experience

In the spring of 2000, the state legislature in Virginia passed a new law regulating the nurse practitioner's prescriptive authority. According to Virginia Code 54.1–2957.01, "Prescription of Certain Controlled Substances and Devices by Licensed Nurse Practitioners":

> In accordance with the provisions of this section and pursuant to the requirements of Chapter 33 of this title, a licensed nurse practitioner . . . shall have the authority to prescribe controlled substances . . . as follows: (i) Schedules V and VI . . . on July 1, 2000; (ii) Schedules IV through VI on and after January 1, 2002; and (iii) Schedules III through VI . . . on and after July 1, 2003.

> Nurse practitioners shall have such prescriptive authority upon the provision to the Board of Medicine and the Board of Nursing of such evidence as they may jointly require that the Nurse Practitioner has entered into and is, at the time of writing a prescription, a party to a written agreement with a licensed physician which provides for the direction and supervision by such physicians of the prescriptive practices of the nurse practitioner. Such written agreements shall include the controlled substances the nurse practitioner is or is not authorized to prescribe and may restrict such prescriptive authority as deemed appropriate by the physician providing direction and supervision. . . .

> This section shall not limit the functions and procedures of certified registered nurse anesthetists. . . . [69]

In Virginia, as in many states, nurse practitioners had acquired the legal authority to prescribe various schedules of medications. According to the law, the specifics would be left to negotiations between physicians and nursing practitioners working together at the grassroots level. The next hurdles would be to institute board of nursing rather than joint Board of Medicine and Board of Nursing oversight of nursing practice, and to convince the American Medical Association to collaborate in the recognition of an expanded scope of practice (including prescriptive authority) for advanced practice nurses and other nonphysician health care providers rather than oppose such changes. In both negotiations, at the individual practice level and at the organizational level, in Virginia and in other states, it would be a matter of trust.

# Conclusion. Toward a More Equitable System of Health Care

In their recent work *Policy Challenges in Modern Health Care,* some of the nation's leading experts in health care policy call for a more equitable system of health care in the United States. Among other things, these policy analysts call for a reduction in barriers to care and the enactment of laws to reduce disparities. And, in chapter 12 of that work, "Improving Quality through Nursing," Professor Linda Aiken notes the increasing role of nurse practitioners in the provision of care.[1] Despite these calls for policy changes in the US health care system, challenges remain. Specific to nursing, these challenges persist in part because the laws governing nursing practice do not reflect the current reality of that practice, and in part because of continued opposition by organized medicine to an expanded role for nursing with regard to prescriptive authority.[2]

As demonstrated here, for over a century nurses have been providing safe and effective care to impoverished Americans in both cities and towns across the country, providing access to care for those to whom it would otherwise be denied. Although that care varied from place to place, and from one decade to the next as new drugs became available and new laws controlling practice were enacted, the nurse's work often included dispensing and furnishing drugs. In fact, for decades nurses held de facto prescriptive authority even as they lacked formal recognition of their work. Later, with the certification of nurse practitioners and changes in their scope of prescriptive authority, nurses with advanced education and certification could also prescribe drugs with medical consultation and support (at least in some states). These nurses had the knowledge they needed to provide safe care. Throughout the century, in all cases in which nurses would furnish or prescribe drugs, the profession insisted that they have advanced education (which varied from post-RN courses early in the century to graduate education in the 1990s) in physical assessment, pathophysiology, and pharmacology. They were also mandated to have supervised clinical experience in these areas—the exact number of hours, of course, varied with the specific historic period. What is clear throughout this history is that the "elusive and fine line" between medicine and nursing was fluid, especially in times and places where nurses were particularly needed. Moreover, the boundaries of the discipline expanded and contracted according to the political, social, and economic context of a particular time and place.

According to a recent report in the *American Medical News,* the American Medical Association is once again confronting changes in scope of practice legislation for non-MD providers, citing patient safety and quality of care issues to be addressed. As Myrle Croasdale, the author of one article, noted:

> With 31 states and the District of Columbia expected to face legislation that asks to alter or expand the scope of more than 20 allied health professions this year, organized medicine says it's time to join forces to oppose any changes that jeopardize the health and safety of the public. . . . The effort is particularly important, committee members say, because all of medicine suffers, not just a single state or medical specialty, when the practice of medicine is put into hands without the training to practice it. . . . In 2006, partnership members plan to conduct research comparing allied health practitioners' training and qualifications to that of physician's education and licensing. . . . "Bottom line, our whole position is public protection. Any decision must be in the best interest of patients," said Lisa Robin FSMB [Federation of State Medical Boards] vice president of leadership and legislative services.[3]

Public protection and "decisions in the best interest of patients" are admirable goals. So are increasing access to health care and reducing disparities in the quality of that care. It will be interesting to see if the Scope of Practice Partnership committee includes historical data in its research.

# Notes

## Introduction

1. Ann B. Hamric, "Using Research to Influence the Regulatory Process," *Advanced Practice Nurse Quarterly* 4, 3 (1998): 44–50.

2. Bonnie Bullough, *The Law and the Expanding Nursing Role* (New York: Appleton-Century, 1975).

3. John Warner, *The Therapeutic Perspective: Medical Practice, Knowledge and Identity in America, 1820–1885* (Princeton: Princeton University Press, 1997).

4. Susan Reverby, *Ordered to Care: The Dilemma of Modern Nursing* (Boston: Cambridge University Press, 1987).

5. Rosemary Stevens, *In Sickness and in Wealth: American Hospitals in the Twentieth Century* (USA: Basic Books, Inc., 1989); quote p. 4.

6. Karen Buhler-Wilkerson, *No Place Like Home: A History of Nursing and Home Care in the United States* (Baltimore: Johns Hopkins University Press, 2001).

7. Nancy Tomes, "The Great American Medicine Show Revisited," *BHM* 79 (2005): 627–63.

8. Barbra Mann Wall, *Unlikely Entrepreneurs: Catholic Sisters and the Hospital Marketplace, 1865–1925* (Columbus: The Ohio State University Press, 2005). Virginia S. Thatcher. *History of Anesthesia: with emphasis on the nurse specialist.* (New York, New York: Garland, 1984). Marianne Bankert, *Watchful Care: A History of America's Nurse Anesthetists* (New York: Continuum, 1989).

9. Laura Ettinger, "Nurse-Midwives, the Mass Media, and the Politics of Maternal Health Care in the United States, 1925–1955," *NHR* 7 (1999): 47–66.

10. Judith Rooks, *Midwifery and Childbirth in America* (Philadelphia: Temple University Press, 1997).

11. Mary Breckenridge, *Wide Neighborhoods: A Story of the Frontier Nursing Service* (New York: Harper and Brothers, Publishers, 1952).

12. Emily K. Abel, "We are left so much alone to work out our own problems": "Nurses on American Indian Reservations during the 1930s," *NHR* 4 (1996): 43–64. See also: Mary Ann Ruffing-Rahal, "The Navajo Experience of Elizabeth Forster, Public Health Nurse," *NHR* 3 (1995):173–88.

13. Julie Fairman, and Joan E. Lynaugh,. *Critical Care Nursing: A History* (Philadelphia: University of Pennsylvania Press, 1998). See also Joan E. Lynaugh and Barbara L. Brush, *American Nursing: From Hospitals to Health Systems* (Cambridge and Oxford: Blackwell Publishers, Inc.,1996).

14. Julie Fairman, "Watchful Vigilance: Nursing Care, Technology and the Development of Intensive Care Units," *Nursing Research* 41, 1 (January/February 1992): 56–60. Julie Fairman, "Playing Doctor?: Nurse Practitioners, Physicians,

and the Dilemma of Shared Practice," in *The Long Term View* [no eds.] (Andover, MA: Massachusetts School of Law at Andover, 1999), 27–35.

15. See Julie Fairman, chapter 14: "Delegated by Default or Negotiated by Need?": Physicians, Nurse Practitioners and the Process of Clinical Thinking," in Ellen Baer, Patricia D'Antonio, Sylvia Rinker, and Joan Lynaugh, eds., *Enduring Issues in American Nursing* (Philadelphia: Springer Publishing, 2001), 309–333.

16. *Sermchief v. Gonzales* 660 S.W. 2ⁿᵈ 693 (Missouri 1983), p. 683.

17. Lavinia Lloyd Dock, *Textbook of Materia Medica for Nurses,* 4th ed. (New York: G. P. Putnam's Sons, 1905), preface, 1: "It is in the hope of filling this middle place [between the medical profession and the lay public] that this textbook has been compiled."

18. Isabella C Herb, "Accidents during and following General Anesthesia," *QSAA, AJS* 30, 9 (1916): 297–302; quote p. 301.

19. Mary Breckenridge, "An Adventure in Midwifery," unpublished manuscript, Frontier Nursing Service Collection, Kornhauser Health Sciences Special Collections, University of Louisville, October 1926, 1–8; quote p. 7.

20. Throughout this work, the term preferred by American Indians today, that of "Indian" rather than "Native Americans" is used. The Indian tribes had various ancestries. The Navajo migrated to the Southwestern region of the United States from Canada.

# Chapter One

1. Elizabeth J. MacKenzie, "Report of the Associate Director, Henry Street Visiting Nurse Service," December 15, 1928 to January 15, 1929, LWC, CU, box 46, folder 1.15, 1–3.

2. For more on this subject, see Marilyn S. Blackwell, "Keeping the 'Household Machine' Running: Attendant Nursing and Social Reform in the Progressive Era," *BHM* 74 (2000): 241–64, and Karen Buhler-Wilkerson, "Bringing Care to the People: Lillian Wald's Legacy to Public Health Nursing," *American Journal of Public Health* 83 (1993): 1778–86.

3. Elizabeth J. MacKenzie, Associate Director of HSS Visiting Nurse Service to Ellis M. Black, MD, Chair of the Medical Economic Committee, Westchester Medical Group, Bronx, New York. (Westchester Village was apparently in the Bronx and is not the city of Westchester as it is known today.).

4. MacKenzie, "Report," 1.

5. For an interesting discussion of tenements on the Lower East Side, see *A Tenement Story: The History of 97 Orchard Street and the Lower East Side Tenement Museum* (New York: The Lower East Side Tenement Museum, 2004).

6. LWC, NYPL, box 43, folder 1.7.

7. According to Hitchcock, alcohol sponge baths every hour were "most in vogue." Jane Hitchcock, "Five Hundred Cases of Pneumonia," *AJN* 3 (1902–03): 169–75; quote p.172. Jane Hitchcock was a member of the New York Hospital Alumnae Association and Head Nurse in the Nurses' Settlement, Henry Street.

8. Lillian Wald, *House on Henry Street* (New York: H. Holt and Company, 1915), 40–41.

9. Lavinia L. Dock, "An Experiment in Contagious Nursing," *AJN* 3 (1902–03): 927–933; quote p. 928.

10. Jane E. Hitchock, "Methods of Nursing in Nurses' Settlement," *AJN* 7 (1906–07): 460–63; quote p. 461.

11. Jane E. Hitchcock, "Five Hundred Cases of Pneumonia," *AJN* 3 (1902–03): 169–175.

12. [na], "The Treatment of Families in Which There is Sickness," Xerox of original, LWC, NYPL, reel 29, 13.

13. Lillian Wald, "The Nurses' Settlement in New York," *AJN* 2, 8 (May 1902): 567–73.

14. Ibid., 570.

15. Karen Buhler-Wilkerson, *No Place Like Home: A History of Nursing and Home care in the United States* (Baltimore: Johns Hopkins University Press, 2001), 112.

16. For more on the care provided by HSS to African Americans, see Marie O. Pitts Mosley, "Satisfied to Carry the Bag: Three Black Community Health Nurses' Contributions to Health Care Reform, 1900–1937," *NHR* 4 (1996): 65–82, and Lucy L. Drown, "A Successful Experiment," *AJN* 1 (July 1901): 729–31.

17. R. L. Duffus, *Lillian Wald, Neighbor and Crusader* (New York: Macmillan, 1938), 43. "Summer bowel complaint" was another term for "infantile diarrhea."

18. Buhler-Wilkerson, *No Place Like Home,* 105–107. Care in the ethnic ghettos of New York at the turn of the century was further complicated by numerous social factors, including "tenement intelligence," extreme poverty, and the inability of many immigrants to speak English. "The dispensary was an autonomous, free-standing institution, created in the hope of providing an alternative to the hospital in providing medical care for the urban poor. . . . In New York . . . the city's dispensaries treated . . . 876,000 patients in 1900." Charles E. Rosenberg, "Social Class and Medical Care in 19th–Century America: The Rise and Fall of the Dispensary," *Journal of the History of Medicine and Allied Sciences* 29 (1974): 32–54; quote p. 32.

19. Lillian Wald, "The Nurses' Settlement," Official Reports of Societies, *AJN* 2 (1901–02): 386–87.

20. Ibid., 386.

21. Buhler-Wilkerson, *No Place Like Home,* 110; see also Diane Hamilton, "The Cost of Caring: The Metropolitan Life Insurance Company's Visiting Nurse Service, 1909–1953, *BHM* 63, 3 (Fall 1989): 420.

22. According to a April 3, 1919 *New York Post* article, "Settlement Takes Over a Saloon," LWC, CU, box 46, folder 1.10. See also "Report of the West Side Committee," LWC, CU, box 42, folder 3, and LWC, VCU, reel 14, box 16, folder 15. In this original documentation, the black nurses are referred to as "colored," as was customary at the time. Notes in this folder indicate "five colored nurses" working in the "colored section" of the city.

23. "Report of the West Side Committee," LWC, CU, box 42, folder 3.

24. Buhler-Wilkerson, *No Place Like Home,* 146–48. For further reading on this topic, see chapter 7 of this work. See also LWC, VCU, reel 14, box 16, folder 15, notes on Metropolitan Life Insurance payments for industrial policy-holders

and Diane Hamilton, "The Cost of Caring: The Metropolitan Life Insurance Company's Visiting Nurse Service, 1909–1953," *BHM* 63 (1989): 414–34.

25. Buhler-Wilkerson, *No Place Like Home,* 147.

26. Diane Hamilton, "The Cost of Caring," 414.

27. Metropolitan Life Insurance Company form, LWC, NYPL, reel 29.

28. *Report of the Nurses' Work of the Settlement* (1905), LWC, CU, box 57, folder 1.3. See also Lillian Wald, "The Care of Sick Children in the Home," paper presented to the Academy of Medicine (May 10, 1917): 2, LWC, NYPL, and *Records,* March and April, 1923, LWC, NYPL, reel 29.

29. Ibid.

30. "Henry Street News," LWC, VCU, reel 72, box 60, folder 6.1.

31. Ibid. A report from the HSS Record Office for March 1923 notes that the nurses made 34,240 home visits that month, "From Information Department, Henry Street Settlement," LWC, NYPL, reel 29.

32. Acetalanid was "a powerful depressant to the spinal nerve centers," an analgesic and antipyretic (used with caffeine "to diminish untoward effects"). It was used in the treatment of migraines. From [no author], *Physician's Handy Book of Materia Medica and Therapeutics* (Detroit, Michigan: Nelson, Baker and Co., 1903), 1. This book included classified list of pharmaceutical preparations. See also Philip J. Hilts, *Protecting America's Health: The FDA, Business, and One Hundred Years of Regulation* (New York: Knopf, 2003), 48. These ingredients (including morphine and alcohol) were often packaged as "soothing syrups" and given to infants, for whom the drugs were often fatal (48).

33. William B. McAllister, *Drug Diplomacy in the Twentieth Century: An International History* (London: Routledge, 2000), 17. By 1895 all the states had passed registration laws for physicians.

34. Hilts, *Protecting America's Health,* 53–54. The testing of drugs prior to marketing them was not controlled by law until the Food, Drug and Cosmetic Act of 1938. See also Anne A. J. Anderman, "Physicians, Fads and Pharmaceuticals: A History of Aspirin," http://www.medicine. mcgill.ca/mjm/issues/v02n02/aspirin.html (accessed January 15, 2005), 1–9.

35. It was not until 1922 that Banting, Best, Macleod, and Collip announced the discovery of insulin. Alexander Fleming isolated penicillin in 1928, but it was not used widely in the U.S. until the 1940s. Prontosil (containing sulfanilamide) was introduced in 1935. These drugs and others were prescribed by physicians. For further documentation of drugs prescribed by physicians in this era, see original prescriptions, KC, CNHI, UVA. See also *Handy Book of Materia Medica,* 1903, 318 for the treatment of tuberculosis: "Treat symptoms as they arise on general principles. Patient should 'live outdoors.' Cod liver oil and cough medicine such as "cannabis indica or heroine, hydrocyanic acid and chloroform," could be used.

36. See Susan Reverby, *Ordered to Care: The Dilemma of American Nursing, 1850–1945* (New York: Cambridge University Press, 1987).

37. Albert T. Lytle, "Materia Medica, Pharmacy and Therapeutics," *AJN* 6 (1905–1906): 217–24. Lytle, a physician from Buffalo, New York, was invited to address the semi-annual meeting of the New York State Nurses Association, Niagara Falls (October 17, 1905). No state required a pharmacy school diploma until New York in 1910. The role of the pharmacist was limited by custom and

law to dispensing only, but prior to 1952, when the Durham-Humphrey amendment to the 1938 Food, Drug and Cosmetic Act came into effect restricting discretionary powers of pharmacists, many counseled patients about medications. Gregory Higby, "Pharmacy in the American Century," *Pharmacy Times* 63 (1997): 16–24. Of significance to this work, the early nurse registration laws only mandated the requirements necessary to qualify an individual as a nurse; they did not define the scope of nursing practice.

38. Lytle, "Materia Medica," 224.

39. Lavinia L. Dock, *Text-Book of Materia Medica for Nurses* (New York: G.P. Putnum's Sons, 1892), preface.

40. M. M. Brown, "The Home Medicine Closet," *AJN* 3 (1903–1904): 196–97. Narcotics such as laudanum were kept freely in the home. Laudanum, an alcoholic solution of opium, was first compounded by Paracelsus about 1527. A leading brand, Sydenham's Laudanum, was introduced in England in 1680. The preparation was used widely through the nineteenth century to treat a variety of disorders. In 1905 the U.S. Congress banned opium (www.intheknowzone.com/heroin/history.htm). Patent medicines during this era claimed to cure a variety of ills. For example, Listerine was advertised as an agent that could prevent disease, including tuberculosis (Hilts, *Protecting America's Health,* 83). See also Minnie Goodnow, "Success in Teaching Materia Medica," *AJN* 7 (1906–1907): 703–4; and *Physician's Handy Book of Materia Medicine* (1903), 328. Icthyol, an ointment, was also called ammonium icthyol-sulphonate. Other forms of icthyol were icthyalbin and icthyolodin.

41. Jane Hitchcock, "500 Cases of Pneumonia." *AJN* 2 (1902): 169.

42. Lillian Wald, "The Nurses' Settlement in New York," *AJN* 2, 8 (May 1902): 567–73; quote p. 571.

43. Ibid., 170–71. Presumably these medicines had been prescribed by a physician according to the law in this era.

44. *Physician's Handy Book of Materia Medica,* 303. Bromoform was prescribed by physicians for whooping cough. To treat "sever paroxysms, a little chloroform or amyl nitrate by inhalation" was noted to give relief. See also: Dock, *Materia Medica,* 89.

45    "Notes on Visits," LWC, NYPL, box 35, reel 24.

46. E. Nora Nagle, RN, "The Mustard Pack," *AJN* 25, 6 (1925): 457–58. "Mustard plasters" are also discussed in Mary Clymer's Training School lecture notes, 1888–1889, MCC, CSHN, UPenn. Mary V. Clymer entered the school of nursing at the Hospital of the University of Pennsylvania in 1887 and kept a carefully written set of lecture notes during her training there. See Joan E. Lynaugh, "Moments in Nursing History: Diary of a Nurse," *Nursing Research* 40, 4 (July–August 1991): 254–55.

47. The HSS nurses also visited middle-class patients and families, particularly after the Metropolitan Life Insurance Company sponsored their services in 1909. See Buhler-Wilkerson, *No Place Like Home;* Lillian Wald, "The Treatment of Families in Which There Is Sickness," *AJN* 4 (1904), reprint LWC, NYPL, reel 29, 1–10.

48. Buhler Wilkerson, *No Place Like Home,* 47.

49. Wald, notes, LWC, VCU, folder 15, box 16, reel 14.

50. Of the 29,105 patients the HSS took care of in 1916, only 33 percent of

the calls came from physicians; 30 percent were referred by the Metropolitan Life Insurance Company. Referrals also came from charitable organizations and clergy. Buhler-Wilkerson, *No Place Like Home,* 103.

51. Lillian Wald, "The Care of Sick Children in the Home," *Speech to the Academy of Medicine, Section on Pediatrics,* (May 10, 1917): 2, LWP, NYPL, reel 25 microfilm.

52. Buhler-Wilkerson, *No Place Like Home,* 103.

53. Martha M. Libster, *Herbal Diplomats* (Golden Apple Publications, 2004), 90–91.

54. Brochure, LWC, VCU, reel 98, box 85, 1–2. One-half pound of flaxseed was listed under "Drug Supplies to be ordered for one of the camps run by the HSS nurses: Supply List 1931," LWC, CU, reel 53, folder 1.13.

55. Flaxseed poultices were made of dried ripe seeds of flax ground into a meal. "A flaxseed poultice must be made over a fire . . . the water must be boiling actively when the meal is added. . . . Flaxseed poultices are sedative. They relieve pain and relax spasm." Lavinia L. Dock, *Text-Book of Materia Medica for Nurse,* 7th ed. (New York: G.P. Putnam's Sons, 1921), 83. Hop bags, containing an aromatic volatile oil, resins, an acid, and an alkaloid called lupuline, were used externally for the relief of pain. They were wrung out with water to apply moist heat, or heated through to provide dry heat (198–99). Bernard Fantus, *The Technic of Medication* (Chicago: Press of the American Medical Association, 1926).

56. LWC, NYPL, reel 29, and "Nurses Settlement Bag," *AJN* 6 (1905–1906): 375. Their work was also called "district nursing." See Lillian Wald, "Official Reports of Societies, Nurses' Social Settlements," paper read before the Third Annual convention of the Nurses' Associated Alumnae of the United States, held in New York, May 3–5, 1900; later published in *AJN* 1 (1900–01): 682–83.

57. [na], "Nurses' Settlement District Bag," *AJN* 1 (1900–01): 769–72.

58. Jane E. Hitchcock, "Five Hundred Cases of Pneumonia," *AJN* 3 (1902–03): 169–74; quote p. 173.

59. Dock, *Materia Medica,* (1921), 276.

60. Ibid., 102.

61. George P. Paul, *A Textbook of Materia Medica for Nurses,* 6th ed. (Philadelphia: W. B. Saunders, 1930). See also *Physician's Handy Book of Materia Medica* (1903).

62. "Nurses Settlement Bag," 375. "Fluid extract of cascara sagrada may be used in conjunction with coarse diet and increase exercise in the curative treatment of constipation," 143; Fantus, *Technic of Medication.* A memorandum from Assistant Director of Nurses Jessie Rogers, RN, to Lillian Wald, December 20, 1920, notes that in a break-in of the Morningside Nursing Office between 6:45 PM, December 19, and 7:00 AM, December 20, "the nurses' bags had been searched" and "two hypodermic syringes" had been taken. She also noted that "the bags were very much disturbed and bottles of solution etc. were thrown about." LWC, CU, box 46, folder 1.10.

63. Lillian Wald, initialed notes (circa 1895, no date on original), LWC, VCU, reel 14, box 16, folder 1, 14. "The loan closet . . . without which no district nurse can work. . . . In it she keeps sheets, blankets, nightgowns, bed linens, rubber sheets . . . syringes, toys, picture books. . . . From it and the medicine chest

the nurse fills her bag. . . . Thermometer, instrument case, swabs, towels, antiseptics solutions, bandages etc."

64. See Dock, *Materia Medica.*

65. Inventory of camp drug supplies, 1931, LWC, CU, box 53, folder 1.13.

66. Dock, *Materia Medica,* 209

67. Ibid., 144.

68. Ibid., 137.

69. Schedule C: "HSS Nursing Expenses," July 31, 1915, LWC, CU, box 57, folder 1.3. See also "Drugs and Supplies, 1935." In the year ending July 31, 1935, drugs and supplies cost $1,026.80 and were a significant proportion of their annual expenses.

70. Dock, *Materia Medica,* 22.

71. Mary Clymer papers, Lecture Notes, December 2, 1888, MCC, CSHN, UPenn. Amyl nitrate is also discussed in *Physicians Handy Book,* 19. It was an "antispasmodic, reducing arterial tension." It was used chiefly by inhalation to relax spasm, notably in asthma and whooping cough. Ergot was used post-partum to "control internal hemorrhaging—particularly uterine" (*Physician's Handy Book,* 63).

72. Ibid.

73. Lillian Wald, "A Social Policy in the Field of Health and Nutrition," (speech at Columbia University, July 2, 1921): reel 25. See also Lillian Wald, "Notes from the Field, 1919," original, LWC, CU, box 46, folder 1.10.

74. According to Margarete Sandelowski, "nurses were trained and expected to collect, record and interpret information vital to the diagnosis without making any claim to participating in diagnosis." Margarete Sandelowski, "The Physician's Eyes: American Nursing and the Diagnostic Revolution in Medicine," *NHR* 8 (2000): 3–38.

75. *Report of a Day in the Work of a Visiting Nurse,* 25 July (c. 1910), LWC, VCU, microfilm reel 98, box 85; Philip C. Jeans and Winifred Rand, *Essentials of Pediatrics for Nurses* (Philadelphia: J. B. Lippincott, 1938), 198. According to Lavinia Dock, *Materia Medica for Nurses,* 7th ed. (New York: G.P. Putnam's Sons, 1921), 221–22, bismuth "acts as a mild sedative and astringent . . . it is given internally as an astringent." According to *Physician's Handy Book,* 29, "Bismuth was used for its "antiseptic action" and "soothing effect on mucus membranes of the stomach." Borax, the common name for "sodium borate, was an antiseptic, "chiefly used for its local action in gargles of the throat. . . ." *Physician's Handy Book* (1903), 132–33.

76. Ira S. Wile, MD, "The Relation of the Public Health Nurse to the Practicing Physicians: The Viewpoint of the Physician," *American Journal of Public Health* (1924): 106–11; quote p. 109.

77. See Sandelowski, "The Physician's Eyes." Wald's notes on district nursing support the autonomy of nurses' practice: the nurse should be "alert and deft in many kinds of services, quick to detect and ready to act, for in this work the doctor is remote and often never seen." Article XII: Registration of Nurses, April 24, 1903. Public Health Law relative to the practice of nursing, Section 206, 599, 126th Session, Laws of New York.

78. Article XII: Registration of Nurses, April 24, 1903. Public Health Law relative to the practice of nursing, Section 206, 599, 126th Session, Laws of New York.

79. Wald, handwritten notes, LWC, NYPL, reel 14, box 15, folder 1. See also

Julia C. Stimson, *Nurses Handbook of Drugs and Solutions,* 4th ed. (Boston: Whitcomb and Barrows, 1925), preface, iv.

80. Lytle, "Materia Medica," 220.

81. *Henry Street Settlement Department of Nursing Booklet,* regulations, LWP, NYPL, reel 29, 3.

82. Notes, "HSS Visiting Nurses," LWP, NYPL, reel 24, box 35, 9.

83. Lillian Wald, "The Treatment of Families in Which There Is Sickness," *AJN* 4 (1904): 9–13.

84. H. P. Hynson, "The Moral and Legal Responsibility of Nurses in the Purchase and Prescribing of Medicines," *AJN* 6 (1905–1906): 290–96. Hynson was a professor at Maryland College of Pharmacy.

85. Edna Foley, "Standing Orders," *AJN* 13 (March 1913): 452. "Standing orders are those orders for treatment and medication, endorsed by the local medical society, which can be used until a physician can be secured or when orders have not been left by the attending physician." National Organization for Public Health Nursing, *Manual of Public Health Nursing* (New York: Macmillan, 1927), 25.

86. "Draft Code of Ethics," January 1926, in correspondence from Elizabeth Fox, President, to the Board of Directors, on the topic. "The Relations of the Nurse to the Medical Profession," LWC, VCU, reel 98, box 85, folder 3. See also correspondence from Lillian Wald to Secretary of the Rockefeller Foundation Jerome D. Green, November 26, 1916, in which Wald speaks of the cooperative efforts of nurses and physicians during the polio epidemic, noting that the doctors were inclined to have children "come to clinic for diagnosis and occasional supervision in order that they may describe to the nurse the muscles they wish exercised or any other treatment that they may care to prescribe." LWC, VCU, reel 106, box 91, microfilm.

87. Fantus, *The Technic of Medication,* 90.

88. Clara Weeks Shaw, *Textbook of Nursing* (New York: D. Appleton, 1902), 298.

89. Fantus, *The Technic of Medication,* 93.

90. Lina L. Rogers, "The Nurse in the Public School," *AJN* 5 (1905): 764–73. In 1904 the staff was increased to 38 nurses which allowed them to cover 100 schools in greater New York (769). Later, physicians made routine inspections only once a month. (769). See also Lina Rogers, "Some Phases of School Nursing," *AJN* 8 (1908): 966. "The New York Board of Health first considered the extension of the already existing system of medical inspection of public schools, by the establishment of a corps of nurses in October 1902" (966).

91. Lina L. Rogers, "School Nursing in New York City," *AJN* 3 (1903): 448–50; quote p. 449.

92. Lina L. Rogers, "Daily Report to Nurses Settlement" (October, c. 1920s), LWC, NYPL, reel 25.

93. Lina L. Rogers, "A Year's Work for the Children in New York Schools," *AJN* 4 (1906): 181–84; quote p. 182.

94. LWC, reel 14, box 16, folder 9. See also Rogers, "A Year's Work." In order to keep children in school and prevent truancy, nurses treated children in school and returned them to the classroom. According to Rogers, an HSS school nurse, "instead of being sent out of school, he is taken to the nurse who promptly wash-

es the sore spot with a tincture of green soap and water and applies a coating of flexible colloidion. After this kind of treatment for a few days the "ring" disappears entirely (182). According to Fantus in *The Technic of Medication,* a 1–2 percent solution of silver nitrate was used to treat trachoma. It was applied by means of a cotton-wrapped application to the everted eyelids. Immediately after the application, the part was irrigated with a physiologic solution of sodium chloride.

95. Wald, untitled original notes on school nursing, reel 32, NYPL, circa 1902. See also Lina L. Rogers, "School Nursing in New York City," *AJN* 3 (1903): 448–50.

96. Rogers, "A Year's Work," *AJN* (1904): 181–84.

97. Lavinia Dock to Lillian Wald, February 1, 1905, LWC, CU. Miss Maude Banfield, Superintendent of Nurses at Graduate Hospital, Philadelphia who was very active in the profession, attended the 1904 International Congress of Nursing meeting (Joan Lynaugh personal communication).

98. Editor's Miscellany, "New Work of the Nurses' Settlement," *AJN* 12 (December 1912): 243–44. This report notes the opening of the third HSS First Aid Room, this one in the Italian Quarter.

99. Dock to Wald, 1 February 1905. It is unclear from the primary sources when the HSS instituted standing orders. However, by 1913, articles appear in the nursing literature about their necessity in public health. See, for example, Foley, "Standing Orders," 452.

100. Obituary, "Dr. Kaplan, Friend of East Side Dies," newspaper article [source unknown] January 7, 1918, LWC, CU, box 49, folder 1.11. One physician to whom the HSS nurses referred patients was Dr. Harry Horner of 77 Park Ave. (LWC, reel 14, box 15, folder 10, 1). Other physicians with whom they worked were "eminent pediatricians Abraham Jacobi, Henry D. Chapin and Henry Koplik." Wald notes for speech on "Nurses and Nursing," LWP, NYPL, reel 25, c. 1930;

101. Letters from Chapin, Jacobi and Koplik, LWC, VCU, reel 25. See also references to Dr. Harry Lorner, 77 Park Ave and referrals for "blood tests" to Dr. Lollis Greenwald, 110 E. 36th Street and Dr. Marcus A. Rothschild, 975 Park Ave. LWC, VCU, reel 14, box 15, folder 10.

102. Buhler-Wilkerson, *No Place Like Home;* Buhler-Wilkerson, "The Call to the Nurse: Our History from 1893–1943," http://www.vnsny.or/mh_about_hist_more.html. *Questions,* vol. 30, no 3 (no further identification of source), 1930, reprint, LWC, NYPL.

103. Bylaws of the Executive Committee of the HS Visiting Nurse Service, LWC, CU, box 42, folder 6, 3.

104. McKensie, "Report of the Associate Director," 1.

# Chapter Two

1. Agnes McGarrell, official reporter, Superior Court California. July 1934. Transcript on Appeal, vol. I. In the Supreme Court of the State of California. *William V. Chalmers-Francis, William Dewey Wightmann, George P. Waller Jr., and Anesthesia Section of the Los Angeles County Medical Association (Plaintiffs) v. Dagmar A. Nelson and St. Vincent's Hospital (Defendants),* Los Angeles Supreme

Court of Appeals No. 364130 (1934), 95–345. Xeroxed copy RG 08113, American Association of Nurse Anesthetist's Executive Office, Historical Files (hereafter cited as AANA, HF). Chicago, Illinois.

2. Ibid.

3. Author telephone conversation with historian of nursing Joan Lynaugh RN, PhD, FAAN, Professor Emerita, University of Pennsylvania, October 4, 2005.

4. For a complete discussion of women's roles, see Catherine Clinton, *The Plantation Mistress: Woman's World in the Old South* (New York: Pantheon, 1982), and Catherine Clinton, *The Other Civil War: American Women in the Nineteenth Century,* 2nd ed. (New York: Hill and Wang, 1999).

5. See for example: Quincealea Brunk, "Caring without Politics: Lessons from the First Nurses of the North and South," *NHR* 2 (1994): 119–36.

6. For a comprehensive overview of the work of Catholic sisters in nursing, see Barbra Mann Wall, *Unlikely Entrepreneurs: Catholic Sisters and the Hospital Marketplace, 1865–1925* (Columbus: The Ohio State University Press, 2005).

7. Catherine S. Lawrence, a Union nurse, reported in her autobiography that she "tied arteries and administered chloroform." Catherine S. Lawrence, *Sketch of Life and Labors of Miss Catherine S. Lawrence* (Albany: James B. Lyon Publisher, 1896), 114. The religious Sisters administered anesthesia at West Pennsylvania Hospital in Pittsburg. E. Jolly, *Nuns of the Battlefield* (Providence, RI: The Providence Visitor Press, 1927), 119. For further reading on this topic, see Barbra Mann Wall, *Unlikely Entrepreneurs,* and Virginia S. Thatcher, *History of Anesthesia with Emphasis on the Nurse Specialist* (Philadelphia: Lippincott, 1953). See also George W. Adams, *Doctors in Blue: The Medical History of the Union Army in the Civil War* (Baton Rouge: Louisiana Paperback edition, 1996); and Sister Mary D. Maher, *To Bind up the Wounds: Catholic Sister Nurses in the U.S. Civil War* (Baton Rouge: Louisiana State University Press, 2005).

8. Also see Wall, *Unlikely Entrepreneurs.*

9. For more on this topic see Susan Reverby, *Ordered to Care* (Boston: Cambridge University Press, 1987).

10. Nancy Harris and Joan Hunziker-Dean, "Florence Henderson: The Art of Open–Drop Ether," *NHR* 9 (2001): 159–84.

11. www.aana.com/archives/timeline.asp (accessed May 12, 2003). See also Wall, *Unlikely Entrepreneurs,* 93.

12. www.aana.com/archives/timeline.asp (accessed May 12, 2003).

13. Nancy A. Harris, "The Administration of Anesthesia—a longitudinal and comparative analysis of Isabel H. Robb's chapter on anesthesia" (paper presented, American Association of the History of Nursing Annual Conference, Atlanta, GA, September 24, 2005). See also Florence A. McQuillen, correspondence to Sister Mary Arthur Schramm, CRNA, PhD, February 21, 1972. McQuillen, who served as executive director of the AANA (1948–1970), related that she had spent two months giving anesthesia in nurses' training. She later worked as a nurse anesthetist at the Mayo Clinic.

14. The Mayo Clinic evolved from the practice of Dr. William Worrall Mayo and his sons, William J. and Charles H. Mayo. It started after a tornado swept through Rochester Minnesota in 1883 when nuns of St. Frances, a Catholic teaching order, were recruited as nurses. In 1889 the Drs. Mayo joined with the nuns

to open a twenty-seven bed hospital which was known as St. Mary's. It was officially labeled the "Mayo Clinic" in 1914. http://www.mayoclinic.org/about/history.html (accessed October 6, 2005).

15. Jean Pougiales, "The First Anesthetizers at the Mayo Clinic," *JAANA* 38, 3 (June 1970): 235–41; quote p. 236.

16. Ibid., 236.

17. Ibid.

18. www.aana.com/archives/timeline.asp (accessed January 16, 2005, p.1).

19. Alice Magaw, "Observations of 1092 Cases of Anesthesia from January 1, 1899 to January 1, 1900," *The St. Paul Medical Journal* 2 (May 1900): 306–311; quote p. 307.

20. Ibid., 308.

21. Other noted women anesthesiologists include Virginia Apgar, MD and Gertie F. Marx, MD. Isabella Herb also had a certificate of pharmacy. She developed the Department of Anesthesiology at what became Rush-Presbyterian Hospital in Chicago, Illinois. Robert Strickland, "Isabella Coler Herb, MD: An early leader in anesthesiology," *Anesthesia and Analgesia* 80, 3 (March 1995): 600–605. http://gateway.ut.ovid.com/gw2/ovidweb.cgi. (accessed July 7, 2005). Isabella C. Herb, "Observations on One Thousand Consecutive Cases of Anesthesia in the Service of Dr. A. J. Ochsner, Augustana Hospital," *Chicago Medical Recorder* 15 (1898): 397–403.

22. Pougailes, "The First Anesthetizers," 239.

23. Ibid.

24. Florence Henderson, "The Nurse as Anesthetist," *AJN* (1909): 947–54; quote p. 948. Henderson worked for the Mayo physicians until 1917.

25. Agnes McGarrell, official reporter, Superior Court of California (July 1934). Transcript on Appeal, vol. I. In the Supreme Court of the State of California. *William V. Chalmers-Francis, William Dewey Wightmann, George P. Waller Jr., and Anesthesia Section of the Los Angeles county Medical Association (Plaintiffs) v. Dagmar A. Nelson and St. Vincent's Hospital (Defendants).* L.A. SC of Appeals No. 364130 (1934): 155–170. Xeroxed copy RG 08113, AANA, HF, Chicago, Illinois.

26. Ernest Sachs, MD, Professor Clinical Neurological Surgery, Washington University School of Medicine, St. Louis, Missouri, "Banquet Speaker," NANA, 1 October 1935, Hotel Chase, St. Louis. Published in *The Bulletin of National Association of Nurse Anesthetists* 4, 1 (January 1936): 38–42.

27. Magaw, "Observations on 1092 Cases," 309.

28. Henderson, "Nurse as Anesthetist," 947.

29. Ibid., 949.

30. Lorrie A. Bennett, CRNA and Barbara A. Jerabek, CRNA, "Sophie Gran Jevne Winton: A Woman and Nurse Anesthetist before Her Time, April 24, 1887 to April 24, 1989" (master's thesis, Mayo School of Health Related Sciences, Rochester Minnesota, 1999), AANA, HF.

31. Magaw, "Observations on 1092 Cases," 306.

32. Alice Magaw, "A Review of Over Fourteen Thousand Surgical Anesthesias," *Surgical Gynecology and Obstetrics* 3 (October 1906): 795–99.

33. Ibid., 797.

34. Frances Truckey, "Anesthesia and Anesthetics," *AJN* 11 (1911): 803–806;

quote p. 803. Truckey, a nurse anesthetist, read this paper before the Toledo Graduate Nurses Association, Toledo, Ohio, April 25, 1911. This continued to be a theme. See also Alice Magaw, "A Review of 14,000 Surgical Cases," *Bulletin of the American Association of Nurse Anesthetists* 7, 2 (May 1939): 66–68.

35. Irvin D. Metzger, MD, "The Nurse as an Anesthetist," *Bulletin of the National Association of Nurse Anesthesia* 11, 3 (1936): 135–38; quote p. 136. Metzger was addressing the fifth annual meeting of the Pennsylvania Association of Nurse Anesthetists, held in Pittsburgh, Pennsylvania, April 23, 1936 and recounted the early years.

36. Robert Stickland, "Isabella Coler Herb, MD: An Early Leader in Anesthesiology," *Anesthesia and Analgesia* 80, 3 (1995): 600–605.

37. Isabella C. Herb, "Administration of General Anesthetics with Special Reference to Ether and Chloroform," *JAMA* 56 (1911): 1312–15.

38. Isabella C. Herb, "Accidents during and following General Anesthesia," *QSAA, AJS* 30, 9 (1916): 297–302.

39. Ibid.; quote p. 297.

40. Magaw, "Observations on 1092 Cases," 306–311; quote p. 308.

41. The next year the speech was published. Herb, "Accidents," 297–302.

42. [na], Society Proceedings, "Interstate Association of Anesthetists," *AJN,* Anesthesia Supplement 30, 10 (1916): 131–32; quote pp. 131–32.

43. Ibid.

44. *Frank v. South,* 175, Ky. 416, 194, S.W. 375 (1917).

45. www.aana.com/archives/timeline.asp (accessed January 16, 2005, p. 1).

46. Deborah Stoner, "Nell Bryant, WWI Nurse Anesthetist," AANA, HF (1999), 1–24.

47. Ibid., 7.

48. Ibid., 8.

49. Ibid., 12.

50. Mary T. Sarnecky, *A History of the U.S. Army Nurse Corps* (Philadelphia: University of Pennsylvania Press, 1999), 130.

51. Bennett and Jerabek, "Sophie Gran Jevne Winton," 9. See also Sarnecky, *A History of the U.S. Army Nurse Corps* for further information on this subject.

52. Hoeffer McMechan, MD (ed.), "Editorial," *AJS, AS* 30 (July 1916): 90.

53. Florence Henderson, "Observations Drawn from an Experience of Twenty-two Thousand Surgical Anesthesias," paper read before the L.A. County Medical Society (June 14, 1917). Published in the *Southern California Practitioner* 32, 10 (October 1917): 154–58.

54. Deborah Stoner, *Nell Bryant, WWI Nurse Anesthetist,* AANA, HF (1999): 14.

55. McMechan, "Editorial," *AJS, AS,* 90.

56. Stoner, *Nell Bryant.* See also McMechan, "Editorial." McMechan notes that "the supply of Novocain [*sic*] is almost at the vanishing point in this country [USA]." On page 90 he notes that the drug was being used in Europe at the front. Meanwhile, the French surgeons used the Gwathney technic of ether-oil colonic anesthesia, especially for operations of the head, face, and neck.

57. Mary T. Sarnecky, *A History of the U.S. Army Nurse Corps* (Philadelphia: University of Pennsylvania Press, 1999), 130.

58. Ibid., 131.

59. Virginia S. Thatcher. *History of Anesthesia: With Emphasis on the Nurse Specialist* (New York: Garland, 1984), 101.

60. In 1927 McQuillen went to the Mayo clinic where she worked for Dr. Charles Mayo. Later, she recalled that during those years the team "experimented with many barbiturates—Amytal, Embutal, Nembutal, and eventually Pentothal." http://www.aana.com/archives/imagine/1996/12imagine96.asp (accessed May 12, 2003).

61. Ohio Statute—Ohio Medical Practice Act, Section 1286–2, (August 2, 1927), (108v. PT., 1, 131). Reprint, AANA, HF.

62. California Pacific Medical Center, "Pioneers: Arthur E. Guedel, MD, 1883–1956, Biography." http://www.cpmc.org/professioanls/hslibrary/collections/guedel/guedelbio.html (accessed October 6, 2005).

63. Bennet and Jerabek, *Sophie Gran Jevne Winton,* 14.

64. Ibid.

65. Thatcher, *History of Anesthesia.*

66. Metzger, "The Nurse as an Anesthetist," 137.

67. Florence A. McQuillen, http://www.aana.com/archives/imagine/1996/12imagine96.asp p. 4 of 6 (accessed May 12, 2003).

68. Brief of National Association of Nurse Anesthetists, Amicus Curiae. In the Supreme court of the State of California. L. A. No. 15162. p. 2. AANA, HF.

69. "Proceedings of the First Annual Meeting of the National Association of Nurse Anesthetists," Milwaukee, Wisconsin, September 13–15, 1933. AANA, HF.

70. The NANA represented about 1200 nurse anesthetists at the time. Virginia S. Thatcher, *A History of Anesthesia with Emphasis on the Nurse Specialist* (Philadelphia: J. B. Lippincott, 1953).

71. Agnes McGarrell, official reporter, Superior Court California. July 1934. Transcript on Appeal, Vol. I. In the Supreme Court of the State of California. *William V. Chalmers-Francis, William Dewey Wightmann, George P. Waller Jr., and Anesthesia Section of the Los Angeles County Medical Association (Plaintiffs) v. Dagmar A. Nelson and St. Vincent's Hospital (Defendants).* L.A. SC of Appeals No. 364130 (1934): 95–345. Xeroxed copy RG 08113, AANA, HF, Chicago, Illinois.

72. Ibid.

73. "Findings and Fact and Conclusion of Law in Recent Nurse-Anesthetist Decision," *Western Hospital Review* (September 1934): 11.

74. *Chalmers-Frances v. Nelson,* California, 1936.

75. Brief of National Association of Nurse Anesthetists, Amicus Curiae. In the Supreme Court of the State of California. L. A. No. 15162. pp. 1–2. AANA, HF.

76. Ibid., 2.

77. *Chalmers-Frances v. Nelson,* California, 1936.

# Chapter Three

1. Betty Lester RN, interview by Jonathan Field, March 3, 1978, #780H146FNS06, transcript p. 1, FNSC, UK-SC, Lexington, Kentucky. Betty Lester was assistant field supervisor for the FNS. Her clinic was located at Bob Fork.

2. In 1928 the manual was titled *Routine for the Use of the Frontier Nursing*

*Service* (hereafter cited as *FNS Routines* [1928]. Later editions were titled *Medical Routines for the Use of the Frontier Nursing Service* (hereafter cited as *FNS Medical Routines*). The manuals were further divided into two sections: (1) *Midwifery Routines* and (2) *Medical Routines, general section. FNS Routine (1928),* box 27, folder 1, FNSC, UK-SC.

3. For the most part, the mountaineers were descendents of the English, Welsh, and Scotch-Irish settlers of the Atlantic seaboard. They had migrated inland to this region. They were often referred to as "Highlanders." Mary B. Willeford PhD, *Income and Health in Remote Rural Areas: A Study of 400 Families in Leslie County Kentucky* (New York City: FNS Inc. 1932), 15–18.

4. See for example: Alexander J. Alexander MD correspondence to Mary Breckenridge, July 10, 1948. Alexander J. Alexander MD was the chairman of the Kentucky Committee for Mothers and Babies in 1927 as noted on the Stationary of the Kentucky Committee (July 12, 1927), FNSC, UK-SC, box 344, folder 1. See also Oral Interview 790H1136 FNS 43 with Edward and Louise Ray, FNSC, UK-SC. Dr. Edward Ray began medical practice in Lexington in 1929.

5. See, for example, the introductions to the *Medical Routines,* 1928, 1936, 1948, etc., FNSC, UK-SC.

6. Mary Willeford, *Income and Health.* For a complete description of the inception and growth of the FNS, see Mary Breckenridge, *Wide Neighborhoods: A Story of the Frontier Nursing Service* (New York: Harper and Brothers Publishers, 1952). See also: Nancy Dye, "Mary Breckenridge, The Frontier Nursing Service and the Introduction of Nurse-Midwifery in the United States," *The Bulletin of the History of Medicine* 57 (Winter 1983): 485–507.

7. Mary Willeford, *Income and Health,* 11.

8. Ibid., 71.

9. See, for example, *Bulletins of the State Board of Health of Kentucky, 1922–1937.* Works Progress Administration (WPA) Series, 11–85, KHSLSC-UL.

10. Susan Allen, "History of the Frontier Nursing Service," http://www.uky.edu/ Libraries/Special/oral_history/Fnshistory.html. (accessed August 15, 2001). The Breckenridge family had a distinguished record of public service. Mary Breckenridge's grandfather had been Vice President of the United States and her father served as foreign minister to Russia.

11. [na]. "Some Specialists: Mary Breckenridge, RN, Nurse-Midwife," *AJN* 30, 3 (March 1930): 311–314.

12. Mary Breckenridge, "Midwifery in the Kentucky Mountains: An Investigation in 1923," reprinted from *The Quarterly Bulletin of the Frontier Nursing Service, Inc.* 17, 4 (Spring 1942): 21–27; quote p. 24.

13. Ibid.

14. For a complete discussion of the show-casing of nurse-midwifery in the United States, see Nancy Dye, "Mary Breckenridge, the Frontier Nursing Service."

15. Winefred Rand RN, "Impression of a Public Health Nursing Service in the Kentucky Mountains," *AJN* 29, 5 (May 1929): 527–30. See also: Mary Breckenridge, "An Adventure in Midwifery," original manuscript (October 1926), 5, KHSLSC-UL, and Mary Breckenridge, *Wide Neighborhoods: A Story of the Frontier Nursing Services* (Lexington: University Press of Kentucky, 1981). The first two [nurse-midwives], Fred Coffin and Edna Rockstroth, were former mem-

bers of the Maternity Center Association in New York and had gone to London to obtain training in midwifery. Breckenridge, "An Adventure in Midwifery," 5.

16. Laura Ettinger, "Nurse-Midwives, the Mass Media, and the Politics of Maternal Health Care in the United States, 1925–1955," *NHR* 7 (1999): 47–66.

17. "Creation of the Bureau," *Five Decades of Action for Children* (Washington DC: United States Department of Health, Education and Welfare Social Security Administration, 1962 reprint), 1. Lillian Wald of the Henry Street Settlement was instrumental in the establishment of the Children's Bureau.

18. Frederick J. Taussig, "The Nurse-Midwife," *PHQ* 6 (June 1914): 33–39.

19. Ibid.

20. Judith Rooks, *Midwifery and Childbirth in America* (Philadelphia: Temple University Press, 1997). See also: Judith W. Leavitt, *Women and Health in America: Historical Readings,* 2nd ed. (Madison: The University of Wisconsin Press, 1999). Later, "As midwives came under state regulation beginning in the early 1920s, they developed a working relationship with public health nurses who were responsible for midwife training campaigns to 'modernize' midwifery." Susan L. Smith, "White Nurses, Black Midwives, and Public Health in Mississippi, 1920–1950," *NHR* 2 (1994): 29–49; quote p. 31.

21. Anna Rude MD, "The Sheppard-Towner Act in Relation to Public Health," *JAMA* 20, 12 (September 16, 1922): 959–64; quote p. 959. Rude was director, Division of Hygiene, United States Children's Bureau. It is interesting to note that Mary Breckenridge refused any federal aid and relied solely on private funding for the FNS.

22. For a complete discussion of the history of childbirth in America, see: Judith Leavitt, *Brought to Bed: Childbearing in America, 1750–1950* (Oxford: Oxford University Press, 1986). See also: Sylvia Rinker, "To Cultivate a Feeling of Confidence: The Nursing of Obstetric Patients, 1890–1940," *NHR* 8 (2000): 117–142, and Sylvia Rinker, "The Real Challenge: Lessons from Obstetric Nursing History, *Journal of Obstetric, Gynecologic, and Neonatal Nursing* 29, 1 (2000): 100–106.

23. Susan Smith, "White Nurses, Black Midwives," 30–31

24. Della Gay, interview by Dale Deaton, September 8, 1978, interview #790H19, transcript pp. 8 and 15, FNSC, UK-SC. Della Gay was a young woman living in Leslie county in the 1920s.

25. Annie Veech, MD, "Child Health Work in Kentucky" (original document, 1922): 1. KHSLSC-UL. And Annie Veech, "But Children Need Mothers," *Child Health Section* Original manuscript (apparently a draft for the newspaper), May 1, 1932, KHSLSC-UL.

26. Willeford, "Income and Health," 38–39.

27. Ibid.

28. Edwin Harper, MD, "Then and Now," *FNS Quarterly Bulletin* 64, 3 (1969): 6. Harper worked at the FNS as a volunteer physician one summer when he was an intern.

29. The work was modeled on the famous Queens nurses of Great Britain, particularly upon the development in the Scotch Highlands, where economic, racial, and geographic conditions were similar. *New York Times,* September 5, 1932, "Kentuckians Greet New Type of Nurse"; Breckenridge, *Wide Neighborhoods;* Rand, "Impressions of a Public Health," 527–30. According to one

report, "Two [of the] nurses, graduates of the Army School and trained in public health at Teachers College and Henry Street, are now taking their midwifery in premier schools of the old world . . . at their own expense." Breckenridge, "An Adventure in Midwifery," 5.

30. Mary Breckenridge, "An Adventure in Midwifery." The nurses were also to follow the rules of the Central Midwives Board (CMB) as far as possible under the conditions in which they worked. Each nursing center was required to keep a copy of the CMB rules and *Fairbairn's Midwifery* text on hand. *FNS Routine* (1928), 10.

31. Chapter 91a. Act of 1914–52. "Nurses–Trained," *The Kentucky Statutes,* 5th ed., vol. 2 (Louisville Kentucky: The Baldwin Law Book Company, 1915): 1934. This law remained in effect, essentially unchanged (except for the extension of the required course of instruction to three years in 1916) until 1950 when it was amended to include a definition of the "Practice of Professional Nursing" which stated: the "Practice of Professional nursing means the practice of nursing by a person who for compensation or personal profit performs any nursing service requiring the application of principles of the biological, physical or social sciences and nursing skills in the care of the sick, in the prevention of disease or in the conservation of health." See *Acts of the General Assembly, The Commonwealth of Kentucky,* chapter 183, S.B. 176. Section 1. Definitions and Application 2b. p. 690.

32. Bonnie Bullough, "The Current Phase in the Development of Nurse Practice Acts," *SLLJ* 28 (1985): 365–95. "By 1923, all the states then in the Union, plus the District of Columbia and Hawaii, had statutes providing for the licensure of nurses" (370). It was not until 1955, when the ANA defined the scope of practice for nursing that this became the model for nurse practice acts in many states.

33. http://www.druglibrary.org/schaffer/Library/studies/cu/cu8.html (accessed August 6, 2004), p. 2.

34. *Frank v. South,* 175, Ky. 416, 194, S. W. 375 (1917).

35. Other physicians included: Marmaduke Brown, Waller Bullock, S. B. Marks, Francis Massie, J. F. Owen, John Scott, and F. Carlton Thomas. Medical Advisory Committee, *Medical Routine for Use of the Frontier Nursing Service* (Lexington, Kentucky, August 27, 1928), preface.

36. *FNS Routines* (1928), 1.

37. Vanda Summers RN, "Saddle-bag and Log Cabin Technic," *AJN* 38, 11 (1938): 1183–84. Vanda Summers, RN, SCM, was one of the British nurse-midwives, trained at the University College Hospital, London. She was working with the FNS when she wrote this article.

38. Oral interview by Carol Crowe Carraco with Molly Lee, February 9, 1979, accession # 790H49FNS58, #56, p.15, FNSC, UK-SC.

39. Summers, "Saddle-bag," 1183–88; quote p. 1183.

40. *FNS Routine* (1928), 10

41. Ibid.

42. The definition used in this book for "to give drugs according to standing orders" is "to furnish." "Proprietary" medicines were "trademarked, patented or secret," according to *Gould's Medical Dictionary* (Scott, 1926) in Willeford, "Income and Health" (1932), 46.

43. *Frank v. South* (1917).

44. *FNS Routine* (1928), 48.

45. See "Contents of Delivery Bag," FNSC, UK-SC, box 225, folder 11.

46. *FNS Routines* (1928), 5–6.

47. *FNS Routines* (1936), 13.

48. *FNS Routines* (1928), 6. See also: Bernard Fantus. *The Technic of Medication* (Chicago: Press of the AMA, 1926), 90. (In this era, both nurses and physicians used these as therapeutic treatments. Prescriptions for these therapies can be found in both the nurses' textbooks and the AMA's publication on prescriptions for physicians; see ch. 2.)

49. *FNS Routines* (1928), 3–8.

50. Mary Breckenridge correspondence to Josephine Hunt MD, December 10, 1925. FNSC, UK, box 344, folder 1.

51. *FNS Routines* (1928), 5–6.

52. Ibid., 20.

53. Florence Nightingale, *Notes on Nursing: What It Is and What It Is Not, Commemorative Edition* (Philadelphia: J. B. Lippincot, 1992; original publication, 1859).

54. For further reading on this topic, see Davinia Allen, "The Nursing-Medical Boundary: A Negotiated Order?" *Sociology of Health and Illness* 19, 4 (1997): 498–520.

55. *FNS Routines* (1928), 28.

56. Ibid., 29.

57. Mary B. Willeford, RN PhD, "Organization and Supervision of the Field Work of the FNS, Inc," *Quarterly Bulletin of FNS* (Summer 1936). FNS, UK-SC, box 25, folder 3.

58. Summers, "Saddle-bag," 1184.

59. Mary Breckenridge, "Yarb Lore in the Kentucky Moutains," *FNS Quarterly Bulletin* (1959): 3–17.

60. Ibid., 12

61. Ibid., 17.

62. Ibid., 7.

63. *FNS Routines* (1928), 5.

64. Breckenridge, "Yarb Lore," 12

65. Ibid., 8

66. Ibid., 15.

67. Ibid., 17.

68. *FNS Medical Routine* (1930), 9.

69. Michael R. Grey, *New Deal Medicine: The Rural Health Programs of the Farm Security Administration* (Baltimore: The Johns Hopkins University, 1999), 21–22. According to Willeford's report: "July 1, 1930 to July 1, 1931 was one of severe drought." Willeford, "Income and Health," 13.

70. Mary Breckenridge, "Corn Bread Line," *Survey* 64 (August 15, 1930), 12.

71. "Kentucky Frontierswomen," draft of original article for the *New York Times,* May 13, 1931. Box 610, 75 KHSL-SC, UL.

72. Mary B. Willeford, "Organization and Supervision of the Field Work of the FNS, Inc," *Quarterly Bulletin of FNS* (Winter 1935): 7–8. The fee for prenatal, delivery and postnatal care was $5.00. A fee of $1.00 was charged per family/year for all other care for those who could pay. In the first 1000 cases, the

FNS nurses had two maternal deaths, both due to chronic heart disease. In the second thousand deliveries, they had no maternal deaths from any cause whatsoever."

73. Ibid.

74. Della Gay interview.

75. Ibid., 21.

76. *FNS Medical Routines* (1936), 1. FNSC, UK-SC, box 27, folder 3.

77. Charlotte Duggar RN, "Letters from a Frontier Hospital," Reprint, *Quarterly Bulletin* 15, 4 (Spring 1940): 2. FNSC, UK-SC, box 25, folder 6.

78. FNS, *Delivery Bag Contents*. FNSC, UK-SC, box 225, folder 11.

79. *FNS Medical Routines* (1936), 28.

80. Ibid., 28.

81. Oral interviews: #19, p. 8; #232, p. 5; #100, p. 7. FNSC, UK-SC, Oral History Project. See also "Trisulfa and Trisulfin" (July 10, 1948), FNSC, UK-SC, box 197, folder 5, and Alexander J. Alexander, MD correspondence to Mary Breckenridge, July 10, 1948. Alexander J. Alexander, MD was the chairman of the Kentucky Committee for Mothers and Babies in 1927 as noted on the Stationary of the Kentucky Committee (July 12, 1927), box 344, folder 1.

82. "Standing Orders," original document about Penicillin orders, FNSC, UK-SC, box 225, folder 11.

83. Alexander J. Alexander correspondence to Mary Breckenridge, July 10, 1948, FNSC, UK-SC, box 334, folder 1.

84. *FNS Medical Routine* (1948), 3

85. "Standing Orders," original document. FNSC UK-SC, box 225, folder 11 (circa 1940–1950s, when Penicillin was widely available in these forms).

86. Mary Willeford, Annual Report 1934. FNSC,UK-SC, box 25, folder 3.

87. Dorothy Buck RN, "Nurse on Horseback Ride On," *AJN* 40, 9 (September 1940): 993–95; quote p. 993.

88. Ibid. See also Nancy Dye, "Mary Breckenridge, the Frontier Nursing Service."

# Chapter Four

1. Elizabeth Forster correspondence to Emily, December 3, 1931. Original correspondence published in "Elizabeth W. Forster and Laura Gilpin," edited by Martha A. Sandweiss, *Denizens of the Desert: A Tale in Word and Picture of Life among the Navajo Indians* (Albuquerque: University of New Mexico, 1988), 54–55. The cough syrup was usually elixir of terpin hydrate and contained alcohol.

2. Elizabeth Forster graduated from the nursing program at Baltimore's Union Memorial Hospital in 1912 and subsequently from an advanced course in public health nursing at Johns Hopkins. Forster, born in 1886 to an old southern family in South Carolina, was forty-four years old at the time that she worked with the Navajos. She had joined the Colorado Springs Visiting Nurse Association in 1913 and became supervisor in 1915, so she had years of experience as a Public Health Nurse prior to her field nursing work in the 1930s. Emily K. Abel, "'We are left so much alone to work out our own problems': Nurses on American

Indian Reservations during the 1930s," *NHR* 4 (1996): 43–64. See also: Mary Ann Ruffing-Rahal, "The Navajo Experience of Elizabeth Forster, Public Health Nurse," *NHR* 3 (1995):173–88.

3. Sandweiss, *Denizens,* Introduction, 9.

4. Ibid.

5. Ibid. E. R. McCray, was the agency superintendent for the region—in Ship Rock. (No first name is given.)

6. Sandweiss, *Denizens,* Introduction, 11–12.

7. Ruth Raup, "The Indian Health Program from 1800 to 1955," NAU-CL, Manuscript (hereafter cited as MS) 269, box 3, folder 217: 7; quote 2.

8. Ibid., 2.

9. Ibid., 6. Earlier, in 1909, funds had been specifically targeted for the treatment of trachoma, however this was the first appropriation for general medical services.

10. United States Public Health Service (USPHS). *Contagious and Infectious Diseases among the Indians,* Senate Document #1083, 62nd Congress, 3rd Session, (Washington, DC: Government Printing Office, 1913), 1–85.

11. Raup, "The Indian Health Program," appendix.

12. Ibid., 5. See also Robert Trennert, *White Man's Medicine: Government Doctors and the Navajo, 1863–1955* (Albuquerque: University of New Mexico Press, 1998), 94.

13. Lewis Meriam, *The Problem of Indian Administration,* (hereafter cited as *The Meriam Report* (Baltimore: The Johns Hopkins Press, 1928), 595.

14. Ibid., 250.

15. Holly T. Kuschell-Haworth, "A History of Federal Indian Health Care," http://academic/udayton.edu/Health/02 organ/Indian03.htm. (accessed July 8, 2005), p. 2 of 5. The New Mexico Association of Indian Affairs was a group organized in Sante Fe in 1922 to represent the political interests of the Pueblo Indians.

16. For a complete discussion of the Navajo beliefs, see Lori Arviso Alvord and Elizabeth C. Van Pelt, *The Scalpel and the Silver Bear: The First Navajo Woman Surgeon Combines Western Medicine and Traditional Healing* (New York: Bantam Books, 2000; quote p. 41. See also: Mary Ann Ruffing-Rahal, "The Navajo Experience of Elizabeth Forster, Public Health Nurse," *NHR* 3 (1995):173–88.

17. *The Meriam Report,* 20.

18. Ibid.

19. [na], "General Information on Nursing in the Indian Health Service (HIS)," April 1928. NAU-CL, MS #269, box 1, folder 10.

20. Ibid., General Information

21. *The Meriam Report,* 192. Lewis Meriam was a 1909 graduate of the George Washington Law School.

22. Ibid., 201.

23. Raup, "The Indian Healt Program," 21.

24. *The Meriam Report,* 16.

25. Charles J. Rhoads was appointed as US Commissioner of Indian Affairs in 1929 by President Herbert Hoover. Rhoads was "a devoted member of the society of Friends and active in Philadelphia area business and academic communities." He had knowledge of Indian problems because of the interests of his father, James E. Rhoads, who helped establish the Indian Rights Association." In http://www.amphisoc.org.

(accessed August 18, 2005). See also: "A Chronicle History of IHS," p. 5. http://academic/udayton.edu/Health/02organ/Indian03.htm (accessed July 8, 2005). "Appropriations earmarked specifically for general health services to Indians began with $40,000 in fiscal year 1911 and grew to almost $18 million in fiscal year 1955. An appropriation of $12,000 for trachoma control work in fiscal year 1910 is sometimes described as the first health appropriation of any significant amount." Raup, "The Indian Health Report," 7.

26. *The Meriam Report,* 258–59.

27. These requirements changed in the 1940s with the shortages due to WWII. Mary Zillitas and Delores Young (who enlisted in the IHS in 1945) were new graduates when they began. See Indian Health Service Nursing Questionnaires (hereafter cited as IHSNQs), NAU-BBWC, MS 269, NAU.PH. 92.14, box 1.

28. Elinor D. Gregg, "News, U. S. Indian Service," *AJN* (May 1933): 507.

29. Ibid.

30. Obituary, Ida E. Bahl, Xerox copy. NAU-BBWC. Ida retired in 1958.

31. See IHSNQ to Ida Bahl, NAU-BBWC, box 7.

32. Department of the Interior, Office of Indian Affairs, "Circular of Information," NAU-BBWC, MS 269, box 1, folder 1.4 (September 1927), 2.

33. Emily K. Abel and Nancy Reifel, chapter 26: "Interactions between Public Health Nurses and Clients on American Indian Reservations during the 1930s," in Judith Leavitt, *Women and Health in America,* 2nd ed., 489–507. According to these authors, the field nurses arrived knowing little or nothing about the Indians and their language and clearly "acknowledged the dominance of white medical knowledge" (quote p. 501).

34. Both Mary Zillitas and Delores Young wrote of this desire for adventure in the IHSNQs, NAU-BBWC, MS 269, box 1.

35. *The Meriam Report,* 249.

36. Ibid.

37. The Navajo had been scattered throughout the Four Corners Region and in 1863, many hid in Canyon de Chelly to escape the invasion of Kit Carson for the US government. During what the Navajo later referred to as "The Long Walk," along 300 miles to Fort Sumner New Mexico, about 200 Indians died. In 1868 the Navajo were allowed to return to what would become the Navajo reservation. www.logoi.com/note/long_walk.html. 4/20/2006.

38. See "Field Nurses' Narrative Reports," NARA, RG75, E779, box 9, [no folders].

39. Laura Gilpin, *The Enduring Navaho (*Austin: University of Texas Press, 1974), 19.

40. Mollie Reebel, "Field Nurse's Narrative Report, April 1933," NARA, RG75, E779, box 9, [no folders].

41. Elizabeth Forster to Laura Gilpin, August 1, 1932. Sandweiss, *Denizens,*102.

42. Elizabeth Forster to Emily, February 20, 1932. Sandweiss, *Denizens,* 70.

43. Gladys Solveson, "Field Nurse's Narrative Report, March 1936," NARA, RG75, E779, box 9, [no folder]. Solveson was a nurse in the Western Navajo Area, Tuba City.

44. Dorothy Williams, "Field Nurse's Narrative Reports, February and March, 1936," NARA, RG75, E779, box 9, [no folders].

45. Mary Eppich, "Field Nurse's Narrative Report, March 1935," NARA, RG75, E779, box 9, [no folder]. Eppich practiced in Shiprock, New Mexico.

46. Lillian B. Watson, "November Narrative report 1955," NAU-BBWC, MS 269, box 1, folder 1.3. For more on their transportation, see *The Meriam Report,* 250. "Lillian Watson began her nursing career in 1955 at Fort Wingate, New Mexico after graduating cum laude from Catholic University in Washington, DC. She initially joined the IHS because there was an acute shortage of trained personnel. In addition to her work at Fort Wingate, Watson taught at the Regina School of Nursing in Albuquerque, New Mexico. After receiving her MSN with honors from the University of California in 1962, she worked in the VISTA program from 1965–1966. In 1973 she became Chief Area Nurse at Windowrock, Arizona, working with the Navajo tribe." From NAU-BBWC, MS 269, Introduction to the collection, p. 3.

47. Mary Zillitas, "Last Navajo Assignment," original manuscript. NAU-BBWC, MS 269. Incoming correspondence to Bahl. box 1, folder 1.4.

48. Abel, "We are left so much alone," to work out our own problems," 49.

49. Mary Zillitas, IHSNQ, NAU-BBWC, box 1, folder 1.4.

50. Mary Eppich, "Field Nurse's Narrative Report, January 1935," NARA, RG75, E779, box 9, [no folders].

51. Mary Eppich, "Field Nurse's Narrative Report, May 1935," NARA, RG75, E779, box 9, [no folders]. Eppich also noted in that report that "the two clinics were held" that month, so apparently she conducted them alone. She had also "treated 66 patients, dispensed 29 medicines," and made "thirteen Hogan calls." This was not always the case, as later, Eppich wrote that Stevenson "made five Hogan calls" with her.

52. Dorothy Loope, IHSNQ to Ida Bahl, 1974. NAU-BBWC. MS 269, box 1, folder 1.4.

53. Mary Eppich, "Field Nurse's Narrative Report, April 1935," NARA, RG75, E779, box 9, [no folders]. Eppich goes on to discuss three other cases in which the "children had symptoms of Tuberculosis." Dr. Elliot confirmed her diagnosis.

54. See Field Nurses' Narrative Reports, NARA, RG75, E779, box 9, [no folders].

55. Ida E. Bahl, "Nurse among the Navajos, 1953–1978," original manuscript (1978). NAU-BBWC, box 1, folder 1.23.

56. Nena Seymour, "Field Nurse's Narrative Report, May 1935," NARA, RG 75, E779, box 9, [no folders].

57. Ruth Seawright. IHSNQ, NAU-BBWC, MS 269, box 1, folder 5.

58. Elizabeth Forster, "Field Nurse's Narrative Report, April 1933," NARA, RG75, E779, box 9, [no folders].

59. Nena Seymour, "Field Nurse's Narrative Report, May 1935," NARA, RG 75, E779, box 9, [no folders].

60. Lillian G. Watson, "Annual Narrative Report, March 1955 to July 1956," original manuscript, NAU-BBWC, MS 269, box 1, folder 1.3.

61. Dorothy Williams, "Field Nurse's Narrative Report, May 1931," NARA, RG 75, E779, box 9, [no folders]. Williams also noted that she visited 22 hogans.

62. Nena Seymour, "Field Nurse's Narrative Report, May 1935," NARA, RG75, E779, box 9, [no folders].

63. Mary Eppich, "Field Nurse's Narrative Report, March 1935," NARA, RG75 E779, Box 9, [no folders]. Eppich practiced in Shiprock, New Mexico. For further reading on silver nitrate, see Stella Goostray, *Drugs and Solutions for Nurses,* 2nd ed. (New York: The Macmillan Co., 1929), 55.

64. Ibid.

65. Mollie Reebel, "Field Nurse's Narrative Report, April 1933," NARA, RG75, E779, box 9, [no folders].

66. Mary Eppich, "Field Nurse's Narrative Report, April 1935," NARA, RG75, E779, box 9, [no folders], 1. Catarrhal fever was a head cold character-ized by "catarrh"—an increase in secretions from mucous membranes. See also Cara Weeks Shaw, *Textbook of Nursing,* 3rd ed. (New York: D. Appleton and Co., 1902).

67. Eppich, "Report, April 1935." See also *Physician's Handy Book of Materia Medica and Therapeutics* (Detroit: Nelson, Baker, and Co., 1903).

68. Lavinia L. Dock, *Textbook of Materia Medica for Nurses* (New York: G. P. Putnam's Sons, 1921), 258.

69. Eppich, "Report, March 1935."

70. Ibid.

71. Ibid. Argyrol was "an organic silver preparation . . . for inflammation of mucus membranes.[or] as a prophylaxis for opthalmia neonatorum." Goostray, *Drugs and Solution,* 57.

72. *Physician's Handy Book of Materia Medica and Therapeutics* (Detroit: Nelson, Baker, and Co., 1903).

73. Dock, *Textbook of Materia Medica for Nurses,* 287.

74. The use of Sulfamide and its derivatives was widespread in the United States by 1939. Perrin H. Long MD, "Sulfamides and Its Derivatives," *AJN* 39, 7 (1939): 719–27. Penicillin was beginning to be used in the early 1940s. Chester S. Keefer MD, "Penicillin," *AJN* 43, 12 (1943): 1076–78. See also: Barbara Brodie, "The Search for Penicillin," *Windows in Time* (Newsletter of the Center of Nursing Inquiry, University of Virginia) 12, 2 (November 2004): 6–8 and 11. "By the spring of 1942, American commercial firms were producing enough Penicillin for research testing. The first intravenous dose of Penicillin was given in March 1942" (p. 8).

75. Elizabeth Forster to Laura Gilpin, January 10, 1932. Sandweiss, *Denizens,* 65.

76. Mary Eppich, "Field Nurse's Narrative Report, December 1935," NARA, RG75, E779, box 9, [no folders]. No first names could be found for these physi-cians in her documentation.

77. Ibid.

78. Gladys Solverson, "Field Nurse's Narrative Report, April 1936," NARA, RG 75, E779, box 9, [no folder].

79. Mollie Reebel, "Field Nurse's Narrative Report, April 1933," NARA, RG75, E779, box 9, [no folders].

80. Lydia T. King, "Field Nurse's Narrative Report, April 30, 1936," NARA, RG75, E779, box 9, [no folders]. King practiced in the Navajo Agency, Klagetoh District. She visited 102 patients that month and dispensed "62 medicines to individuals in field and office."

81. See for example: Mary Eppich, "Field Nurse's Narrative Report, January 1935," NARA, RG75, E779, box 9, [no folders].

82.  Dr. Charles S. McCammon to Ida Bahl, April 1, 1974. NAU-BBWC, MS 269, box 1, folder 1.4.

83.  Emily K. Abel and Nancy Reifel, chapter 26: "Interactions between Public Health Nurses and Clients on American Indian Reservations during the 1930s," in Judith Leavitt, *Women and Health in America,* 2nd ed. (Madison, WI: University of Wisconsin Press, 1999), 489–507.

84.  Delores Young, IHSNQ, NAU-BBWC, box 2, folder 1.4.

85.  Zillatas, IHSNQ, NAU-BBWC, box 1, folder 1.4.

86.  *The Meriam Report,* 88.

87.  Lori Arviso Alvord, MD, and Elizabeth C. Van Pelt, *The Scalpel and the Silver Bear* (New York: Bantum Books, 1999); see also: Mary Zillatas, IHSNQ, NAU-BBWC.MS 269, box 1, folder 1.4.

88.  Sings often involved the use of sandpaintings, elaborate artwork made from various dried sands. See Mark Bahti, *A Guide to Navajo Sandpaintings* (Tucson, AZ: Rio Nuevo Publishers, 2000) for further reading on this topic.

89.  Alvord and Van Pelt, *Scalpel and the Silver Bear,* 186.

90.  Ibid., 6.

91.  Ida E. Bahl, *Nurse among the Navajos,* Part I, Chapter IX. Original manuscript (1978): 62–63.

92.  Dorothy Williams, "Field Nurse's Narrative Report, August 1935," NARA, RG 75, E779, box 9, [no folders]. Williams practiced in the Shiprock District.

93.  Lillian Watson, RN graduated cum laude with a BSN from Catholic University in 1955, and received her Masters of Science in Nursing from the University of Colorado. In the 1960s, she assumed the job of Chief, Area Nursing Service Branch, Navajo Area Indian Health Service, Window Rock, and Arizona. NAU-BBWC, MS 269, box 1. See also: Lillian Watson, "Narrative, November 1955," NAU-BBWC, MS 269, box 1, folder 1.3.

94.  Mary Eppich, "Field Nurse's Narrative Report, April 1935," NARA, RG 75, E779, box 9, [no folders], 2. See also Dorothy Williams, "Field Nurse's Narrative Report, June 1935," NARA, RG 75, E779, box 9, [no folder].

95.  Gladys Solveson, "Field Nurse's Narrative Report, March, 1936," NARA, RG 75, E779, box 9, [no folder].

96.  Robert Trennert, *White Man's Medicine: Government Doctors and the Navajo, 1863–1955* (Albuquerque: University of New Mexico Press, 1998), 33.

97.  Gladys Solveson, Field Nurse's Narrative Report, March 1936. NARA, RG75, E779, box 9, [no folder].-

98.  Dorothy Williams, "Field Nurse's Narrative Report, February 1936," NARA, RG75, E779, box 9, [no folders].

99.  Emily K. Abel and Nancy Reifel, chapter 26: "Interactions between Public Health Nurses and Clients on American Indian Reservations during the 1930s," in Judith Leavitt, *Women and Health in America,* 2nd ed. (Madison: University of Wisconsin Press, 1999), 489–507.

100.  Elizabeth Forster, "Field Nurse's Narrative Report, May 1933," NARA, RG75, E779, box 9, [no folders].

101.  In emergencies, they did deliver babies. Mary Zillitas did an emergency delivery, receiving instructions by telephone. She had to give ergotrate and vitamin K for post-partum hemorrhage and transport the patient 37 miles to a hospital. See Mary Zillitas' record IHSNQ, NAU-BBWC, MS 269.

102. Mollie B. Reebel, "Report, April 1933," p.2.

103. Nena Seymour, "Field Nurse's Narrative Report, August 1935," NARA, RG75, E779, box 9, [no folders].

104. Zillitas, IHSNQs, NAU-BBWC, MS 269, box 1.

105. Nena Seymour, "Field Nurse's Narrative Report, July 1935," NARA, RG75, E779, box 9, [no folders], 2.

106. Delores Young, IHSNQs, NAU-BBWC, MS 269, box 1. Delores worked in 1945 in Crownpoint New Mexico in a hospital and wrote that she "enjoyed the cadet nurses and Red Cross nurses who came to help out."

107. Ibid. Young wrote about taking children to Salt Lake City.

108. Ibid.

109. Raup, "The Indian Health Program," 9.

110. Watson, Annual Report, p. 3.

111. [na], Monthly Narrative 1957, NAU-BBWC, MS 269, box 7, folder 437. TB remained a problem in the 1950s among the Native Americans.

112. Watson, Annual Report, p. 3.

113. Harold Foster, report to Ida Bahl in the 1970s (no title). NAU-BBWC, MS 269, box 1, folder 4.

114. American Nurses Association, "ANA Board Approves a Definition of Nursing Practice," *American Journal of Nursing* 55, 5 (1955): 1474.

115. Arlene Keeling and Jeri Bigbee, "chapter 1: "The History of Advanced Practice Nursing in the United States," In *Advanced Nursing Practice: An Integrative Approach,* Ann Hamric, Judith Spross and Charlene Hanson, eds. (Philadelphia: W. B. Saunders Co., 2005).

## Chapter Five

1. Margene O. Faddis RN, "Eliminating Errors in Medication," *AJN* 39, 11 (November 1939): 1217–23. Faddis, RN, MA, was Associate Professor of Medical Nursing at the Frances Payne Bolton School of Nursing, Western Reserve University, Cleveland, Ohio.

2. Barbara Melosh, *The Physician's Hand: Work Culture and Conflict in American Nursing* (Philadelphia: Temple University Press, 1982).

3. For more on this topic, see Jean Whelan, "Smaller and Cheaper: The Chicago Hourly Nursing Service, 1926–1957," *NHR* 10 (2002): 83–108.

4. Melosh, *The Physician's Hand.*

5. Joan Lynaugh and Barbara Brush, *American Hospitals: From Hospitals to Health Care Systems* (Cambridge, MA: Blackwell, 1996), 36. By the mid-1930s, hospitals had begun to hire graduate nurses to supplement their student-nurse staff. See Melosh, *The Physician's Hand.*

6. Clara Weeks-Shaw, *Textbook of Nursing* (New York: D. Appleton and Company, 1902), 182.

7. The Flexner Report was one of the most important events in the history of American and Canadian medical education. It was a commentary on the condition of medical education in the 1900s and the impetus for major changes in medical education. The report is named after Abraham Flexner, an educator (not a physician), who prepared it for the Carnegie Foundation. For further reading on

this topic see Rosemary Stevens, *In Sickness and in Wealth, American Hospitals in the Twentieth Century* (New York: Basic Books, 1989).

8. Joel D. Howell, *Technology in the Hospital: Transforming Patient Care in the Early Twentieth Century* (Baltimore: Johns Hopkins University Press, 1996).

9. For further reading on this topic, see Stevens, *In Sickness and in Wealth;* Howell, *Technology in the Hospital.*

10. Stevens, *In Sickness and in Wealth,* 105.

11. Michael Bliss, *The Discovery of Insulin* (Chicago: University of Chicago Press, 1984) and Chris Feudtner, *Bittersweet: Diabetes, Insulin and the Transformation of Illness* (Chapel Hill: University of North Carolina Press, 2003).

12. Ibid., 109

13. See Melosh, *The Physician's Hand.* See also Susan Reverby, *Ordered to Care: The Dilemma of American Nursing, 1850–1945* (Boston: Cambridge University Press, 1987).

14. Melosh, *The Physician's Hand.*

15. M. L. Montag and M. Filson, "Administration of Medicines," *Nursing Arts* (Philadelphia: W. B. Saunders, Co. 1948), 482–87.

16. For further reading on this topic, see Susan Reverby, *Ordered to Care;* Melosh, *The Physician's Hand.*

17. Nan H. Ewing, "A Medicine Board," *AJN* 39, 10 (1939): 1086–87.

18. Ibid., 1087

19. Ibid. See also Lavinia L. Dock, *Textbook of Materia Medica for Nurses* (New York: G. P. Putnam's Sons, 1927). Beginning in the Great Depression, the majority of RNs in America were employed by hospitals as staff nurses. They were not working in the Frontier Nursing Service or in migrant camps or on Indian reservations; instead, they worked in hospitals throughout the country—on general medical and surgical wards, in obstetrics, psychiatry, and pediatrics, in operating rooms, and in out-patient clinics. Public Health Nurses did have "standing orders," at least in 1912 in Chicago. See Edna Foley, RN, "Standing Orders," *AJN* 13 (1913): 451–53.

20. This phenomenon was later described by a psychiatrist in the 1960s. See Leonard Stein, "The Doctor-Nurse Game," *Archives of General Psychiatry* 16 (1967): 699–703.

21. For a complete discussion of the idea of new spaces, see Joan Lynaugh and Julie Fairman, "New Nurses, New Spaces: A Preview of the AACN History Survey," *American Journal of Critical Care* 1, 1 (1992): 19–24. See also Julie Fairman and Joan E. Lynaugh, *Critical Care Nursing: A History* (Philadelphia: University of Pennsylvania Press, 1998).

22. Eleanor C. Lambertson, *Nursing Team Organization and Functioning* (New York: Bureau of Publications, Teachers College, Columbia University, 1953).

23. Concern for preventing medication errors was a common theme in the nursing literature. By 1939, Faddis, writing in *AJN,* made a plea for "the exclusive use of white medication cards instead of the colored ones which had long been in use, so that "orders could be more easily read," Faddis, *AJN* 39, 11: 1220. In the same article (p. 1218) she noted "the oft-repeated 'read the label three times' is one of the best ways to prevent errors. . . . If the label is read with care when first the bottle is taken from the shelf, when the drug is removed and again when the bottle is replaced, fewer nurses will have cause for regret."

24. B. Harmer and V. Henderson, eds. "Chapter 25: Administration of Medicines." *Textbook of the Principles and Practice of Nursing*, 5th ed. (New York: The MacMillan Co., 1955), 693–94.

25. Julie Fairman, "Playing Doctor?: Nurse Practitioners, Physicians, and the Dilemma of Shared Practice," *The Long Term View* [no eds.] (Andover, MA: Massachusetts School of Law at Andover, 1999), 27–35.

26. Margene O. Faddis, "New Drugs," *AJN* 41, 7 (July 1941): 759–63. According to Faddis: "sulfapyridine was accepted for inclusion in *New and Nonofficial Remedies* in 1939" (p. 759), while "sufathiazole was synthesized in 1939 and accepted by the council on Pharmacy and Chemistry in January 1941" (p. 760). For further reading on the history of Penicillin see: Barbara Brodie, "The Search for Penicillin," *Windows in Time*, 12, 2 (November 2004): 6–8 and 11.

27. Joel D. Howell, *Technology in the Hospital: Transforming Patient Care in the Early Twentieth Century* (Baltimore: Johns Hopkins University Press, 1996).

28. U.S. Department of Commerce, Bureau of the Census, *Historical Statistics of the United States—Colonial Times to 1970*, Part I (Washington, DC: US Government Printing Office, 1975), 55.

29. Truman, Harry, "Statement by the President on the Toll Taken by Heart Diseases." www.whistlestop.org/50 year_archive/50yr020749_statement.htm. 7 February 1949.

30. Hughes W. Day, "An Intensive Coronary Care Area," *Diseases of the Chest* 44, 4 (1963). Mortality from MI was 30–40 percent.

31. H. Borst and F. Mohr, "History of Coronary Artery Surgery—A Brief Review," *Journal of Thoracic Cardiovascular Surgery* (2001).

32. Ibid. See also Joel D. Howell, "Early Perceptions of the Electrocardiogram: from Arrhythmia to Infarction," *Bulletin of the History of Medicine*, (1984): 58; and Elizabeth Gill, "Some Recent Developments in Drug Therapy," *AJN* 44, 8 (August 1944): 741–44.

33. Headlines: "Lyndon Johnson: Out for This Session," *New York Times*, July 3, 1955.

34. Headline: "Eisenhower is in Hospital with 'Mild' Heart Attack; his condition called 'good,'" *New York Times*, September 25, 1955. For further reading, see: Clarence G. Lasby, *Eisenhower's Heart Attack* (Lawrence: University Press of Kansas, 1997).

35. See Lasby, *Eisenhower's Heart Attack*. Also see: Cover: Photograph of Eisenhower in Wheelchair, *Life Magazine*, November 14, 1955. Story with photos: 71–74. Headline: "President Spends Day without Use of Oxygen Tent," *New York Times*, September 29, 1955.

36. Faye Abdellah and E. Josephine Starchan, "Progressive Patient Care," *AJN* 59, 5 (May, 1959): 649–55.

37. Ibid., 651.

38. Ibid. For further reading on this topic, see Julie Fairman, "Watchful Vigilance: Nursing Care, Technology and the Development of Intensive Care Units," *Nursing Research* 41, 1 (January/February 1992): 56–60. Even during WWII, at home in the United States, the task of starting an IV was still within the domain of medicine.

39. Abdellah and Starchan, *Progressive Patient Care*, 652.

40. William B. Kouwenhoven, James R. Jude, G. Guy Knickerbocker,

"Closed Chest Cardiac Massage," *JAMA* 173 (July 9, 1960): 1064–67; quote p. 1064.

41. James R. Jude, William B. Kouwenhoven, G. Guy Knickerbocker, "Cardiac Arrest," *JAMA* 178, 11 (December 16, 1961): 1063–70.

42. Claude S. Beck, "Resuscitation for Cardiac Standstill and Ventricular Fibrillation Occurring during Operation," *American Journal of Surgery* 54 (October 1941): 273.

43. Claude S. Beck, E. C. Wechesser, and F. M. Barry, "Fatal Heart Attack and Successful Defibrillation," *JAMA* 161, 5 (June 2, 1956): 434–36.

44. Indeed, physicians controlled which medical tasks they delegated to nurses and which tools of the trade nurses could use. From the turn of the twentieth century, doctors had delegated to nurses the tasks of administering oral and intramuscular medications and taking the patient's temperature, pulse rate, and respiration (TPR). They also delegated dressing changes. After completing the initial dressing change of a surgical incision site, a surgeon would expect the nurse to change the consecutive dressings. In order to remove the tape and gauze easily, the nurse would use a special "bandage scissors" to cut the dressing. Because of her responsibility for these three tasks, the thermometer, syringe, and bandage scissors became trademarks of nursing practice. See Margarete Sandelowski, "The Physicians' Eyes: American Nursing and the Diagnostic Revolution in Medicine," *NHR* 8 (2000): 3–38; quote p. 24.

45. Arlene Wynbeek Keeling, "Memoirs of a Student Nurse in Coronary Care," 1969, unpublished paper.

46. Sandelowski, "The Physicians' Eyes," 5.

47. Mildred Crawley, "Care of the Patient with Myocardial Infarction," *AJN* 61, 2 (February 1961): 68.

48. Physicians who would initiate coronary care units were in Australia, Toronto, California, Miami, Kansas City, New York, and Philadelphia.

49. Day, "An Intensive Coronary Care Area," 424.

50. Hughes W. Day, "History of Coronary Care Units," *American Journal of Cardiology* 30 (1972): 405.

51. Hughes W. Day, "An Intensive Coronary Care Area," *Diseases of the Chest* 44, 4 (1963): 424.

52. Judith Stuart, "Hartford Coronary Care Unit," unpublished manuscript, KC, CNHI.

53. Judith S. Jacobson, *The Greatest Good: A History of the John A. Hartford Foundation* (New York: John A. Hartford Foundation, 1984).

54. Presbyterian was a 325-bed institution. Approximately 170 patients were admitted each year with AMI. Lawrence E. Meltzer and J. Roderick Kitchell, Grant Proposal NU00096–01, PC, CNHI.

55. Ibid.

56. Ibid., 6.

57. Ibid.

58. Ibid. 11.

59. Laurence E. Metzger, Rose Pinneo, and Rodderick Kitchell, *Intensive Coronary Care: A Manual for Nurses* (Philadelphia: Presbyterian Hospital CCU Fund, 1965), preface.

60. Rose Pinneo, "Historical Perspectives of Coronary Care Units," speech

given in Chicago, Illinois, June 1981: PC, CNHI. Rose Pinneo received her BA from Maryville College, Maryville, Tennessee, her diploma from Johns Hopkins Hospital, and her MS in Education from the University of Pennsylvania. She was Assistant Educational Director and Medical Nursing Instructor, West Jersey Hospital, Camden, New Jersey, and Medical-Surgical Instructor, University of Pennsylvania. Curriculum Vitae, Rose Pinneo, PC, CNHI. Rose Pinneo, RN, MSN, interview by author, Sebring, Florida, Novembers 19, 1999; transcript in PC, CNHI.

61.  Rose Pinneo, "Mastering Monitoring," *Nursing '72* (1972): 1–4. PC, CNHI.

62.  Pinneo interview, 1999

63.  Rose Pinneo, "Machines in Perspective: Nursing in a Coronary Care Unit," *AJN* 65, 2 (1965): 76–79. See also Janice Lufkin, telephone interview with author, November 13, 2001, transcript in KC, CNHI; and Lynn Warner telephone interview with author, August 20, 2001, transcript in KC, CNHI.

64.  Rose Pinneo, "Nursing Care of the Cardiac Patient," paper presented at the Third Clinical Nursing Conference, sponsored by the AHA Nursing Committee and the ANA Conference Group on Medical-Surgical Nursing, Miami Beach, Florida, October, 1965; PC CNHI, p. 3.

65.  Janice Lufkin, telephone interview with author, November 13, 2001. Transcript KC, CNHI. Lufkin, a 1962 graduate from Presbyterian Hospital School of Nursing, worked for a few months after graduation in the eye and ear ward and then as a graduate nurse in the Maximum Care Unit. She rotated to the new two-bed CCU in January 1963 when it opened. She began to work there full-time and became head nurse after Helen Haugh resigned. In 1966 she left the CCU and entered the navy.

66.  Lynn Warner telephone interview by author, August 20, 2001; transcript in KC, CNHI. Warner, a 1963 diploma graduate of Presbyterian Hospital School of Nursing, worked in the first group of nurses who staffed the Presbyterian CCU. Her previous experience included a year of night shift work in the Maximum Care Unit at Presbyterian. Subsequently, she received a PhD in nursing.

67.  Lufkin interview.

68.  Ibid.

69.  Warner interview. Dilantin was introduced in 1938 for the control of seizures in epilepsy. (See Faddis, "New Drugs.") It was later used as a treatment for cardiac arrhythmias. It had to be mixed in normal saline rather than in Dextrose and water to ensure that it would dissolve. In the 1960s, nurses rather than pharmacists mixed IV solutions and some medicines at the bedside.

70.  Meltzer et al., *Intensive Coronary Care,* 2.

71.  Pinneo, "Mastering Monitoring," 3.

72.  Hughes Day, "An Intensive Coronary Care Area," *Diseases of the Chest* 44 (1963): 423–27, and Thomas Lee and Lee Goldman, "The Coronary Care Unit Turns 25: Historical Trends and future directions," *Annals of Internal Medicine* 108 (1988): 887–94.

73.  Lawrence Meltzer and J. Roderick Kitchell, "The incidence of arrhythmia associated with myocardial infarction," *Progress in Cardiovascular Disease* 9 (1966): 915–27.

74.  http://rmp.nlm.nih.gov/rmp/D/A/A/rmddaa.html. 10/16/05.

75.  Lawrence E. Meltzer, Rose Pinneo, and J. Roderick Kitchell, *Intensive*

*Coronary Care: A Manual for Nurses,* rev. ed. (Philadelphia: Charles Press, 1972), 8.

76. See nurse interviews, Presbyterian Hospital and Bethany Hospital. Transcripts, KC, CNHI.

77. Arlene Keeling, "Memoirs of CCU Nursing, 1960s and 1970s," unpublished paper.

78. Fairman and Lynaugh, *Critical Care Nursing.*

79. Susan M. Reverby, *Ordered to Care: The Dilemma of American Nursing, 1850–1945* (New York: Cambridge University Press, 1987); Davina Allen, "The Nursing-Medical Boundary: A Negotiated Order?" *Sociology of Health and Illness* 19, no. 94 (1997): 498–520.

80. Fairman and Lyanugh, *Critical Care Nursing,* 24.

81. Even in the 1970s, the chief of medicine at the University of Virginia, Edward Hook, MD, did not approve of having "standing admission orders" to the CCU. His argument was that the house staff had to learn what orders to write. Meanwhile the house-staff physician bypassed this problem by writing "CCU routine," thereby allowing nurses to implement care as they usually did. Keeling unpublished memoirs, CCU at the University of Virginia, 1971–1974.

82. Sandelowski, "The Physicians' Eyes." See also Allen, "Negotiated Boundary."

# Chapter Six

1. Robert Isquith, RN, "Pediatric Nurse Practitioner Succeeds Mother as Indian Health Care Provider," *Commitment* 3, 3 (Summer, 1978): 22–26; quote p. 24.

2. Ibid., 22. Durran was part Ute and part Navajo.

3. Ibid., 24.

4. Ibid.

5. Loretta Ford, "A Nurse for All Settings: The Nurse Practitioner," *Nursing Outlook* (August 1979): 516–20; quote p. 517. The four-month didactic section of the curriculum was followed by months of supervised clinical experience.

6. Barbara Brush and Elizabeth A. Capezuti, "Revisiting a Nurse for All Settings": The Nurse Practitioner Movement, 1965–1995," *Journal of the American Academy of Nurse Practitioners* 8, 1 (January 1996): 5. See also Julie Fairman, "Playing Doctor?": Nurse Practitioners, Physicians and the Dilemma of Shared Practice," *The Long Term View* 4 (Andover, MA: Massachusetts School of Law at Andover 1999): 27–35. See also Loretta Ford, "A Deviant Comes of Age," *Heart and Lung,* 26, 2 (March–April 1997): 87–91.

7. Ford, "A Nurse for All Settings," 516–20; quote 517.

8. Ford, "A Deviant Comes of Age," 87–91.

9. Isquith, "Pediatric Nurse Practitioner Succeeds Mother," 24.

10. Julie Fairman, "The Roots of Collaborative Practice: Nurse Practitioner Pioneers' Stories," *NHR* 10 (2002): 159–74; quote 163. Meanwhile, medicine was interested in attracting more doctors to primary care. And in 1969, amid vocal concern about the decline of general practice and rousing calls for new roles for "personal physicians" and "primary care"—medicine made general practice a "specialty" with the formation of the American Board of Family Practice.

11. F. M. Jones, "ANA Certification for Specialization," in J. C. McCloskey and H. K. Grace, eds., *Current Issues in Nursing* (Boston: Blackwell Scientific, 1981).

12. Joan Lynaugh, Patricia Gerrity, and Gloria Hagopian, "Patterns of Practice: Master's Prepared Nurse Practitioners," *Journal of Nursing Education* 24, 7 (September 1985): 291–95; quote p. 291.

13. Ford, "A Deviant Comes of Age," 87.

14. U.S. Congress, House Committee on Interstate and Foreign Commerce, Subcommittee on Public Health and Safety. *Nurse Training Act of 1964.* Hearings before the subcommittee (Washington, DC: Government Printing Office, 1964). See also U. S. Congress, Senate, Committee on Labor and Public Welfare, *Nurse Training Act of 1964.* Report to Accompany H. R. 11241 (Washington, DC: Government Printing Office, 1964): Report no. 1378, 1–24.

15. American Nurses' Association, "Educational Preparation for Nurse Practitioners and Assistants: A Position Paper," *AJN* 65 (1965): 106–11.

16. Ford, "A Deviant Comes of Age," 87. Functional areas of nursing, like administration and education, became minor content areas.

17. Ibid., 88.

18. Loretta C. Ford, "Nurse Practitioners: History of a New Idea and Predictions for the Future," In L. H. Aiken, ed., *Nursing in the 80s* (Philadelphia: J. B. Lippincott, 1982), 231–48.

19. Terrance Keenan, "Support of Nurse Practitioners and Physician Assistants," chapter 11. http://www.rwjf.org/publications/publicationsPdfs/anthology1999/chaper_11.html. (2/19/2004).

20. Ford, "A Deviant Comes of Age," 88.

21. For extensive reading on the Clinical Nurse Specialist, see Ann B. Hamric, "History and Overview of the CNS Role," in A. B. Hamric and Judith A. Spross, eds., *The Clinical Nurse Specialist in Theory and Practice,* 2nd ed. (Philadelphia: W. B. Saunders, 1989), 3–18.

22. Ford, "A Nurse for all Settings," 516–21; quote 517.

23. The history of the process of certification for nurse practitioners is beyond the scope of this work. For more information, see Dr. Julie Fairman's work on the subject. See also: the National Association of Pediatric Nurse Associates and Practitioners collection (hereafter cited as NAPNAP), and the National Certification Board of Pediatric Nurse Practitioners and Nurses papers (hereafter cited as NCBPNP), CNHI, UVA.

24. Martha E. Rogers, "Nursing: To Be or Not to Be," *Nursing Outlook* 20 (1972): 42–46. See Luther Christman, "Advanced Practice Nursing: Is the physician's assistant an accident of history or a failure to act? *Nursing Outlook* 46, 2 (1998): 56–59. For further reading see R. Ballweg, "History of the Profession," chapter 1 in R. Ballweg, S. Stolberg, and E. M. Sullivan, *Physician Assistant* (Philadelphia: W. B. Saunders, 1994), 1–20.

25. Rogers, "Nursing: To Be or Not to Be." See also Joan Lynaugh, Patricia Gerity, and Gloria Hagopian, "Patterns of Practice: Master's Prepared Nurse Practitioners," *Journal of Nursing Education* 24, 7 (September 1985): 291–95, and Reba de Tornyay, "Expanding the Nurses' Role Doesn't Make Her a Physician's Assistant," *AJN* 71, 5 (May 1971): 974–75.

26. J. Moxley, "The Predicament in Health Manpower," *AJN* 68 (1968): 1490.

27. Lynaugh, Gerrity, and Hagopian, "Patterns of Practice," 291–95.

28. Ibid.

29. Christman, "Advanced Practice Nursing," 56–59.

30. Ibid., 56.

31. R. Ballweg, "History of the Profession," chapter 1 in Ballweg et al., *Physician Assistant,* 1–20.

32. Isquith, "Pediatric Nurse Practitioner Succeeds Müther," 25.

33   Lynaugh, Gerrity, and Hagopian, "Patterns of Practice," 291.

34. Loretta Ford and Henry Silver, "The Expanded Role of the Nurse in Child Care," *Nursing Outlook* 15, 8 (1967): 43–45.

35. P. Kalisch and Bernice Kalisch, *The Advance of American Nursing,* 2nd ed. (Boston: Little, Brown and Company, 1986).

36. [na] "Editorial," *AJN* (1971): 53.

37. Denise Geolot, "Federal Funding of Nurse Practitioner Education: Past Present and Future," *Nurse Practitioner Forum* 1, 3 (December 1990): 159–62.

38. Mailings to State Nurse Associations, 1970 New York State Nurses' Association (hereafter NYSNA) archives records on the American Nurses' Association. In Jerelyn P. Weiss, RN, FNP, JD, "Nursing Practice: A Legal and Historical Perspective," *Journal of Nursing Law* 2, 1 (n.d.): 17–35; quote 28.

39. Joan Lynaugh and Barbara Brush, *American Nursing: From Hospitals to Health Systems* (Cambridge, MA: Milbank Memorial Fund and Blackwell Publishers, 1996).

40. Terrance Keenan, "Support of Nurse Practitioners and Physician Assistants," chapter 11. http://www.rwjf.org/publications/publicationsPdfs/anthology1999/chaper_11.html. (2/19/2004), 3 (hereafter cited RWJ).

41. Ibid.

42. Ibid., 4

43. Ibid. The Henry Street Settlement was no longer a viable site for this type of project. The Visiting Nurse Service of the Settlement separated from Henry Street in 1944 to become the Visiting Nurse Service of New York. Henry Street activities focused on social issues since that time. http://www.henrystreet.org/site/PageServer?paagename+abt_history (accessed 10/19/2005).

44. Booz, Allen, and Hamilton, Management consultants [no first names available], "Family Nurse Practitioners in Kentucky," *FNS Quarterly Bulletin* (1970): 3–11. Reprint [no volume or number] in FNS Collection UKSC. At about the same time, an interdisciplinary team led by Richard Kirk, MD at the University of Kentucky also studied the use of nurses to provide primary care in Appalachia and concluded that "formally trained nurse practitioners working as 'physician associates' could increase the effectiveness of our health care system." Richard Kirk, Joseph Alter, Helen Browne, and Judith Davis, "Family Nurse Practitioners in Eastern Kentucky," *Medical Care* 9, 2 (March–April 1971): 160–68.

45. Booz, Allen, and Hamilton, "Family Nurse Practitioners," 5–6.

46. Ibid., 6–7. See also [no author] "A Training Program for Development of the Family Nurse Practitioner," *FNS Quarterly Bulletin* 45, 1 (1970): 34–40.

47. [na], "Frontier School of Midwifery and Family Nursing Celebrates 50th Anniversary 1939–1989," *FNS Quarterly Bulletin* 64, 4 (Spring 1989): 2–7; quote 3.

48. Ibid., 4. In 1977, the FSMFN affiliated with the University of Kentucky College of Nursing. In 1985 it affiliated with Bellarmine College of Louisville and the Frances Payne Bolton School of Nursing at Case Western Reserve University of Cleveland, Ohio. Through these affiliations, students were able to earn graduate credit for courses taken at FNS and apply them towards a Master Degree in Nursing at these institutions.

49. Ira Moscovice, "The Influence of Training Level and Practice Setting on Patterns of Primary Care Provided by Nursing Personnel," *Journal of Community Health* 4, 1 (Fall 1978): 4–14; quote p. 5. See also Gertrude Issacs, "Frontier Nursing Service Continuing Development 1974," *FNS Quarterly Bulletin* 49, 2–3 (Autumn 1973/Winter1974): 3–15.

50. Ibid., 5.

51. [na], "Distribution of Drugs—FNS," typed manuscript, FNS, UKSC (no date, circa 1975), 1–4.

52. Ibid., 1.

53. Ibid.

54. Ibid. Narcotics were considered "controlled" substances and there were specific guidelines for their use outlined in the Harrison Narcotic Act of 1914. Nurses and physicians had to account for each and every dose of such drugs as morphine and codeine. Since the reception of the FNS, Breckenridge had employed young women from well-to-to families to serve as couriers.

55. Ibid. By 1975 the FNS employed four physicians and a pharmacist in addition to the nurses and support personnel. Helen Tirpak, "The Frontier Nursing Service :Fifty years in the Mountains," *Nursing Outlook* 23, 5 (May 1975): 308–10.

56. "Distribution of Drugs," FNSC-UK, 2

57. "In the fiscal year 1976, 70.6 percent of the funded grants were at the certificate level and 23.55 were at the master's level." Denis H. Geolot, "NP Education: Observations from a National Perspective," *Nursing Outlook* 35, 3 (1987): 132–35.

58. RWJ, 6.

59. Geolot, "NP Education," 132.

60. Lynaugh, Gerrity, and Hagopian, "Patterns of Practice," 291.

61. Personal communication of author with Barbara Brodie, RN PhD FAAN, The Madge Jones Professor Emerita, The University of Virginia School of Nursing. 10/17/05. Barbara Brodie had visited Loretta Ford a few years before Brodie accepted a faculty position at the University of Virginia and was very interested in the PNP role.

62. Geolot, "NP Education,"133. Telephone conversation between author and Barbara Brodie, October 17, 2005. See also Barbara Brodie, *Mr. Jefferson's Nurses* (Charlottesville, Virginia: Rector and Visitors University of Virginia, 2001).

63. Lynaugh, Gerrity, and Hagopian, "Patterns of Practice," 291.

64. Arlene Keeling and Jeri Bigbee, chapter 1, "The History of Advanced Practice Nursing in the United States," in Ann B. Hamric, Judith A. Spross, and Charlene M. Hanson, eds., *Advanced Nursing Practice: An Integrative Approach* (Philadelphia: W. B. Saunders, 2005). The Chapel Hill meeting would lay the foundation for the formation of the National Organization of Nurse Practitioner Faculties (NONPF).

65. Fairman, "Playing Doctor," 41–42.

66. Fairman, "The Roots," 163–64.

67. Mary Ann Draye and Marie A. Brown, "Surviving the Proving Ground: Lessons in Change from NP Pioneers," *The Nurse Practitioner* 25, 10 (2000): 60–71; quote 65.

68. Ibid., 67.

69. Fairman, "The Roots," 164. Clearly, the rules were different outside settings like FNS or the Indian Health Service.

70. Author interview with Barbara Dunn, RN, PNP. Richmond, Virginia, 2004.

71. Elizabeth H. Hadley, "Nurse and Prescriptive Authority: A Legal and Economic Analysis," *American Journal of Law and Medicine* 15, 2–3 (1989): 245–99.

72. Ibid., 25.

73. Idaho Code 54–1413, 1971.

74. Barbara J. Safriet, "Health Care Dollars and Regulatory Sense: The Role of Advance Practice Nursing," *Yale Journal on Regulation* 9, 2 (Summer, 1992): 417–88; quote p. 445. Moreover, the Drug Enforcement Act (DEA) required that practitioners wishing to prescribe controlled substances obtain DEA registration numbers, and only those practitioners with broad prescriptive authority (e.g., physicians and dentists) could get these numbers.

75. "The North Carolina legislature first enacted legislation in 1975 that authorized nurse practitioners and physician's assistants to prescribe drugs. 1975 N.C. Session Laws 627 (codified at N.C. Gen. Stat 90–18.1)." Hadley, "Nurses and Prescriptive Authority," 268.

76. See Barbara J. Safriet, "Health Care Dollars," *Yale Journal on Regulation* 9, 2 (Summer 1992): 417–88. See also Ellen Baer, "Philosophical and Historical Bases of Primary Care Nursing," in M. D. Mezey and D. O. McGivern, eds., *Nurses, Nurse Practitioners Evolution to Advanced Practice,* 2nd ed. (Boston: Little, Brown, 1993), 102–116.

77. Vernellia R. Randal, "A Chronological History of IHS," http://academic.udayton.edu/Health/020rgan/Indian02.html. 8 of 10.

78. Fairman, "Playing Doctor," 40. Medicare funds had become available in 1965 under Lyndon Johnson's Great Society legislation.

79. Marlene Heffer, MD, "Monthly Report. April 1979," NAU-CL 313, MS 269, box 7, folder 447.

80. In 1984 an Associate Professor at the University of Wisconsin- Madison, Joy Calkin, proposed a model for "advanced nursing practice," specifically identifying CNSs and NPs with master's degrees as Advanced Practice Nurses (APNs). Ann B. Hamric, Judith A. Spross, and Charlene M. Hanson, eds., *Advanced Nursing Practice: An Integrative Approach* (Philadelphia: W. B. Saunders, 1996).

81. M. Faut-Callahan and M. Kremer, "The Certified Registered Nurse Anesthetist," in A. B. Hamric, J. A. Spross, and C. M. Hanson, eds., *Advanced Nursing Practice: An Integrative Approach* (Philadelphia: W. B. Saunders, 1996), 421–44.

82. Keeling and Bigbee, chapter 1: "The History of Advanced Practice Nursing." The organization would finally succeed in 1989.

83. P. Repicky, R. Medenahall, and R. Neville, "Professional Activities of Nurse Practitioners in Ambulatory Care Settings," *The Nurse Practitioner* 5, 2 (1980): 27–40.

84. Koch, Pazaki, and Campbell, "The First 20 Years," 64. See also Brush and Capezutie, "Revisiting," 5–11.

85. J. Levine, S. Orr, D. Sheatsley, Jake Lohr, and Barbara Brodie, "The Nurse Practitioner: Role, Physician Utilization, Patient Acceptance," *Nursing Research* 27 (1978): 245–54.

86. Koch et al., "The First 20 Years," 65.

87. Bonnie Bullough, "State Nurse Practice Acts," in *Nurse, Nurse Practitioner: Evolution to Advanced Practice,* 3rd ed., revised by Virginia Gillett and Vern L. Bullough (Boston: Little, Brown, 1999): 369–93.

88. William B. Schaffrath, PhD, Director, National Joint Practice Commission, *Statement on Medical and Nurse Practice Acts* (The National Joint Practice Commission, USA, June 6, 1975), 13.

89. Ibid., 14.

90. E-mail correspondence, Kathy H. Haugh to Brenda Stewart, July 10, 2000. re: AMA history about "Resolution H-275–986 ('Our Illustrious History') AMA." The resolution was reaffirmed in 1994 and 1997.

## Chapter Seven

1. E-mail message received by Arlene W. Keeling, RN PhD, Director of the Acute Care Nurse Practitioner Program at the University of Virginia School of Nursing, 2/15/00, p. 1 of 3 [names omitted to ensure confidentiality].

2. Ibid. The landmark 1938 Federal Food, Drug, and Cosmetic Act terminated consumer control over choice of medications, even though such was clearly not the intent of that law. Physicians were chosen as the providers to select medications. Antoinette Inglis and Diane Kjervik, "Empowerment of Advanced Practice Nurse: Regulation Reform Needed to Increase Access to Care," *Journal of Law, Medicine and Ethics* 21, 2 (1993): 193–205.

3. Ibid. See also Safriet, "Health Care Dollars," 457, footnotes 134 and 135.

4. Ibid.

5. Massachusetts Medical Society, "Vital Signs," http://www.massmad.or/AM/Template.cfm?Section=Inside_MMS35&CONTENTID=8 (accessed 10/18/2005), p.1.

6. See Inventory of camp drug supplies, 1931, LWC, CU, box 53, folder 1.13. In 2000, of course, there were many more over-the-counter drugs in Schedule VI (e.g., Ibuprophen, Tylenol PM, Benadryl, hydrocortisone creams, Desitin [for diaper rash], Lotrimin antifungal cream, Digel, Mylanta, etc.). It also included the wide variety of herbal remedies available to the public.

7. E-mail received by Arlene Keeling, RN PhD, Director of the Acute Care Nursing Practicitoner Program at the University of Virginia. Subject: HB 818. 2/18/00, p.1 of 3.

8. Ibid.

9. Emily Couric, correspondence to Joanne Peach FNP, February 13, 2000. Peach Collection (PCH), CNHI.

10. Ibid., 1.

11. Safriet, "Health Care Dollars," 456–57.

12. Hadley, "Nurses and Prescriptive Authority: A Legal and Economic

Analysis," 269. See also North Carolina Session Laws 627 codified in *North Carolina General Statutes* 90–18.1 (1975).

13. Antoinette Inglis and Dione Kjervik, "Empowerment of Advanced Practice Nurse," *Journal of Law, Medicine, and Ethics,* 193–205.

14. *Sermchief v. Gonzales,* 660 S.W. $2^{nd}$ 693 (Missouri 1983), p. 683.

15. E. Doyle, and J. Meurer, "Missouri Legislation and Litigation: Practicing Medicine without a License," *Nurse Practitioner* 8 (1983):41–44.

16. Ibid., 687.

17. Ibid. Amici briefs were letters and documents of support sent to the court stating reasons the judges should decide in favor of one position.

18. Ibid.

19. Ibid., 685.

20. Ibid., 688–90.

21. Ibid.

22. [na], "History and Historical Highlights 1973 through 1998. http://www.nanda.org/html/history1.html 10/21/2005. Conference Proceedings were published following each biannual conference. Editors included Derry Moritz, Mi Ja Kim, Gertrude McFarland, Audrey McLane and Rosemary Caroll Johnson. In 1982 the group incorporated and formed the North American Nursing Diagnosis Association (NANDA). Much has been written on this topic. Further discussion of NANDA is beyond the scope of this work.

23. Hadley, "Nurse and Prescriptive Authority," 251.

24. Lynaugh and colleagues reported that 90 percent of the responses (of NPs in their survey form 1975–1985) noted that they worked in ambulatory settings, "particularly hospital or community based clinics." Joan Lynaugh, Patricia Gerity, Gloria Hagopian, "Patterns of Practice: Master's Prepared Nurse Practitioners," *Journal of Nursing Education* 24, 7 (September 1985): 291–95; quote p. 292.

25. Grace M. Sills, chapter 42: "The Role, Function of the Clinical Nurse Specialist," *The Nursing Profession: A Time to Speak,* N. L. Chaska, ed (New York: McGraw-Hill Book Co, Inc. 1983), 563–79; quote p. 566.

26. Safriet, "Health Care Dollars," 445.

27. See also Ann B. Hamric, Judith A. Spross, and Charlene M. Hanson, eds., *Advanced Practice Nursing: An Integrative Approach,* 3rd ed. (Philadelphia: W. B. Saunders, 2000). These authors have been leaders in the cause to clearly label what is and what is not "advanced practice nursing." The label itself is still being discussed in the profession as a proposed broader definition, the "Doctor of Nursing Practice, or DNP" may replace it.

28. Joy Calkin, "A Model for Advanced Nursing Practice," *Journal of Nursing Administration* 14, 1 (1984): 24–30.

29. Hamric et al., *Advanced Practice Nursing.*

30. H-275–986. From "Resolution ["Our Illustrious History"], AMA. E-mail correspondence, Kathy H. Haugh to Brenda Stewart, July 10, 2000. re: AMA history. The resolution was reaffirmed in 1994 and 1997.

31. Safriet, "Health Care Dollars," 429.

32. Ibid.

33. See Safriet's "Health Care Dollars" for a complete discussion of this issue.

34. Diane F. Mahoney, "Nurse Practitioners as Prescribers: Past Research

Trends and Future Study Needs," *The Nurse Practitioner* 17, 1 (January 1992): 44–51; quote p. 47.

35. Safriet, 461.

36. Ibid.

37. American Medical Association, *Regulation of Prescription-Writing Authority of Nurse Practitioners.*

38. Barbara Bibb, "Comparing Nurse-Practitioners and Physicians: A Simulation Study on Processes of Care," *Evalution and the Health Professions,* 5, 1 (March 1982): 29–42. For further discussion of this topic see: Larry Koch, S. H. Pazaki, and James D. Campbell, "The First 20 Years of Nurse Practitioner Literature: An Evolution of Joint Practice Issues," *The Nurse Practioner: A Journal of Primary Health Care* 17, 2 (February 1992): 62–71.

39. See, for example, Dorothy Brooten, S. Kumar, P. Butts, S. Finkler, et al., "A Randomized Clinical Trial of Early Hospital Discharge and Home Follow-up of Very Low Birth-weight Infants," *New England Journal of Medicine* 315 (1986): 934–39, and S. Brown and D. Grimes, "A Meta-analysis of Process of Care, Clinical Outcomes, and Cost Effectiveness of Nurses in Primary Care Roles: Nurse Practitioners and Nurse Midwives" (Washington DC: The American Nurse Association Division of Health Policy, 1992). It is beyond the scope of this work to review all of the literature on this topic.

40. Office of Technology Assessment, Nurse Practitioners, Physicians Assistants and Certified Nurse Midwives: A Policy Analysis (U.S. Congress, HCS 37, 1986).

41. Mary O. Mundinger RN DrPH, "Twenty-first-century Primary Care: New Partnerships between Nurses and Doctors," *Academic Medicine* 77, 8 (August 2002): 776–80.

42. See Rosemary Stevens, *American Medicine and the Public Interest* (Berkeley and Los Angeles: University of California Press, 1998).

43. Arlene Keeling and Jeri Bigbee, chapter 1: "History of Advanced Practice Nursing," in Hamric et al.

44. *Frank et al. v. South* (1917).

45. *Chalmers-Frances v. Nelson* (1934 and 1936).

46. *Bhan v. NME Hospitals, Inc., et al.* (1985). 772 F.2d 1467 (9th Circuit Court).

47. Donna Diers, "Nurse-midwives and Nurse Anesthetists: The Cutting Edge in Specialist Practice," in L. H. Aiken and C. M. Fagin, eds., *Charting Nursing's Future: Agenda for the 1990s* (New York: J. B. Lippincott, 1991), 159–80.

48. Barbara J. Safriet, JD, "Still Spending Dollars, Still Searching for Sense: Advanced Practice Nursing in an Era of Regulatory and Economic Turmoil," *Advanced Practice Nursing Quarterly* 4, 3 (1998): 24–33; quote p. 25.

49. During the 1960s and 1970s, the other major advanced practice role for nursing was the Clinical Nurse Specialist (CNS), many of whom worked in specialty areas of hospitals, like the CCU, renal units, neurology units, etc. (The nurse anesthetist was already in existence.) During the 1970s, federal funding from the Professional Nurse Traineeship Program provided fiscal support to new graduate programs in nursing for CNSs. Meanwhile, several specialty nursing organizations, including the American Association of Critical Care Nurses

(AACN) and the Oncology Nursing Society (ONS), developed. In addition, the ANA's Congress of Nursing Practice operationally defined the role of the CNS, and nursing began to conduct evaluative research on the outcomes of CNS care. By mid-decade, the American Nurses Association (ANA) officially recognized the CNS role, operationally defining the CNS as an expert practitioner and a change agent. Of particular significance, the ANA's definition included master's education as a requirement for the CNS (ANA, Congress of Nursing Practice, 1974). See Keeling and Bigbee, in Hamric et al, chapter 1, for further reading on the Clinical Nurse Specialist history. The Nurse Training Act of 1964 (Title VIII of the Public Health Service Act, H. R. 10042) provided federal funding for the construction of nursing schools, faculty development, special projects, and student loans and scholarships. Between 1964 and 1971, Congress appropriated more than $334 million for nursing education.

50. Safriet, "Health Care Dollars," 440.

51. Jerome Kassirer, "What Role for Nurse Practitioners in Primary Care?" *The New England Journal of Medicine* 330, 3 (January 20, 1994): 204–205.

52. Ellen D. Baer, "Philosophical and Historical bases of Advanced Practice Nursing Roles," *Nurse, Nurse Practitioners' Evolution of Advanced Practice,* 3rd ed. (Philadelphia: Springer, 1999), 87–88. See also M. Beck, "Improving America's Health Care: Authorizing independent prescriptive privileges for advanced practice nurses," *University of San Francisco's Law Review* 29 (1995): 951.

53. New York State Education Act, Article 139, Section 6902, paragraph 3a, (1995). Paragraph 3b authorizes nurse practitioner's prescriptive powers with similar restraints.

54. Barbara Daly, *The Acute Care Nurse Practitioner* (New York: Springer Publishing Company, 1997).

55. Ann Keane and Therese Richmond, "Tertiary Nurse Practitioners," *Image: Journal of Nursing Scholarship,* 25, 4 (1993): 281–84; quote p. 282.

56. A. Mitchell-DiCenso, G. Guyatt, M. Marrin, R. Goeree, A. Willan, et al., "A Controlled Trial of Nurse Practitioners in Neonatal Intensive Care," *Pediatrics,* 98, 6 (1996): 1143–48.

57. During the second half of the twentieth century, numerous national organizations, including NAPNAP, The Academy of Pediatric Nurse Practitioners, and The National Certification Board of Pediatric Nurses and Practitioners administered certification examinations to NPs. For a complete review of this topic, see Julie Fairman's work on the subject.

58. Ruth Kleinpell, "Acute Care Nurse Practitioners: Roles and Practice Profiles," *American Association of Colleges of Nursing, Clinical Issues* 8, 1 (1997):156–62. See also H. Shah, K. Brutlomesso, D. Sullivan, and J. Lattanzio, "An Evaluation of the Role and Practices of the Acute Care Nurse Practitioner," *AACN Clinical Issues,* 8,1 (1997): 147–55.

59. Jeri Bigbee and A. Amidi-Nouri, "History and Evolution of Advanced Nursing Practice," in Hamric, Spross and Hanson, eds, *Advanced Nursing Practice: An Integrative Approach* (Philadelphia: W. B. Saunders Co., 1996), 3–32.

60. Jerome P. Kassirer, MD, "What Role for Nurse Practitioners in Primary Care?" *The New England Journal of Medicine* 330, 3 (January 20, 1994): 204–205.

61. Ibid.

62. This was certainly the case in the Acute Care Nurse Practitioner program

at the University of Virginia, which had required student and faculty ACNPs to use them since 1998. The use of PDAs was mandated in the other NP tracks in 2001. See University of Virginia News: "School of Nursing Bestows Innovative Teaching Awards" (January 8, 2001). http://www.virginia.edu/topnews/releases2001/schoolofnursing-jan-8–2001.html, (accessed 10/22/2005).

63. Ellen Baer, Chapter 3: "Philosophical and Historical Basis of Advanced Practice Nurse roles," in *Nurse, Nurse Practitioners: Evolution of Advanced Practice* 3rd ed. (1999), 72–91; quote p. 79.

64. During the 1990s, the number of NPs increased dramatically in response to increasing demand, the national emphasis on primary care, and the concomitant decrease in the number of medical residencies in the sub-specialties.

65. National Organization of Nurse Practitioner Faculties (NONPF), *Criteria for Evaluation of Nurse Practitioner Programs* (Washington, DC: National Task Force on Quality Nurse Practitioner Education, 1997). See also American Association of Colleges of Nursing (AACN), *Enrollment and Graduations in Baccalaureate and Graduate Programs in Nursing* (Washington, DC: Government Printing Office, 1999).

66. NONPF, *Criteria.*

67. Leslie Boyd, "Advanced Practice Nursing Today," *Medical Economics* 63, 9 (September 2000): 57–62; quote p. 62.

68. Safriet, "Still Spending Dollars," 24–33; quote p. 25.

69. Virginia Code 54.1–2957.01, "Prescription of Certain Controlled Substances and Devices by Licensed Nurse Practitioners."

# Conclusion

1. David Mechanic, Lynn B. Rogut, and David C. Colby, *Policy Challenges in Modern Health Care* (Rutgers, NJ: Rutgers University Press, 2005).

2. Myrle Croasdale, AMNewsStaff, Feb. 13, 2006 "Professional Issues," (AMA 2006). www.fsmb.org/grpolpolicydocs.html.

3. Ibid., 2.

# Select Bibliography

Abdellah, Faye, and E. Josephine Starchan. "Progressive Patient Care." *American Journal of Nursing* 59, 5 (May 1959): 649–55.

Abel, Emily K. "We are left so much alone to work out our own problems": "Nurses on "American Indian Reservations during the 1930s." *Nursing History Review* 4 (1996): 43–64.

Adams, George W. *Doctors in Blue: The Medical History of the Union Army in the Civil War.* Baton Rouge: Louisiana Paperback edition, 1996.

Allen, Davinia. "The Nursing-Medical Boundary: A Negotiated Order?" *Sociology of Health and Illness* 19, 4 (1997): 498–520.

Alvord, Arviso, and Elizabeth C. Van Pelt. *The Scalpel and the Silver Bear: The First Navajo Woman Surgeon Combines Western Medicine and Traditional Healing.* New York: Bantam Books, 2000.

American Nurses Association. "ANA Board Approves a Definition of Nursing Practice." *American Journal of Nursing* 55, 5 (1955):1474.

_____. "Educational Preparation for Nurse Practitioners and Assistants: A Position Paper." *American Journal of Nursing* 65, 12 (December 1965): 106-111.

Baer, Ellen D. "Philosophical and Historical bases of Advanced Practice Nursing Roles." In *Nurse, Nurse Practitioners' Evolution of Advanced Practice.* 3rd ed. Philadelphia: Springer, 1999, 87–88.

Beck, Claude S. "Resuscitation for Cardiac Standstill and Ventricular Fibrillation Occurring during Operation." *American Journal of Surgery* 54 (October 1941): 273.

Beck, Claude S., E. C. Wechesser, and F. M. Barry. "Fatal Heart Attack and Successful Defibrillation." *Journal of the American Medical Association* 161, 5 (June 2, 1956): 434–36.

Beck, M. "Improving America's Health Care: Authorizing independent prescriptive privileges for advanced practice nurses." *University of San Francisco's Law Review* 29 (1995): 951.

Bennett, Lorrie A., and Barbara A. Jerabek. "Sophie Gran Jevne Winton: A Woman and Nurse Anesthetist before Her Time, April 24, 1887 to April 24, 1989." Master's Thesis, Mayo School of Health Related Sciences, Rochester Minnesota, 1999.

Bibb, Barbara. "Comparing Nurse-Practitioners and Physicians: A Simulation Study on Processes of Care." *Evaluation and the Health Professions* 5, 1 (March 1982): 29–42.

Blackwell, Marilyn S. "Keeping the 'Household Machine' Running: Attendant Nursing and Social Reform in the Progressive Era." *Bulletin of the History of Medicine* 74 (2000): 241–64.

Bliss, Michael. *The Discovery of Insulin.* Chicago: University of Chicago Press, 1984.

Boyd, Leslie. "Advanced Practice Nursing Today." *Medical Economics* 63, 9 (September 2000): 57–62.

Breckenridge, Mary. "Midwifery in the Kentucky Mountains: An Investigation in 1923." Reprinted from *The Quarterly Bulletin of the Frontier Nursing Service, Inc.* 17, 4 (Spring 1942): 21–27.

_____. *Wide Neighborhoods: A Story of the Frontier Nursing Service.* New York: Harper and Brothers Publishers, 1952.

_____. "Yarb Lore in the Kentucky Moutains." *FNS Quarterly Bulletin* (1959): 3–17.

Brodie, Barbara. "The Search for Penicillin," *Windows in Time* (Newsletter of the Center of Nursing Inquiry, University of Virginia) 12, 2 (November 2004): 6–8 and 11.

Brooten, Dorothy, S. Kumar, P. Butts, S. Finkler, et al. "A Randomized Clinical Trial of Early Hospital Discharge and Home Follow-up of Very Low Birth-weight Infants." *New England Journal of Medicine* 315 (1986): 934–39.

Brown, S., and D. Grimes. "A Meta-analysis of Process of Care, Clinical Outcomes, and Cost Effectiveness of Nurses in Primary Care Roles: Nurse Practitioners and Nurse Midwives." Washington, DC: The American Nurse Association Division of Health Policy, 1992.

Brown, M. M. "The Home Medicine Closet." *American Journal of Nursing* 3 (1903–1904): 196–97.

Brunk, Quincealea. "Caring without Politics: Lessons from the First Nurses of the North and South." *Nursing History Review* 2 (Philadelphia: University of Pennsylvania Press, 1994): 119–36.

Buck, Dorothy. "Nurse on Horseback Ride On." *American Journal of Nursing* 40, 9 (September 1940): 993–95.

Buhler-Wilkerson, Karen. "Bringing Care to the People: Lillian Wald's Legacy to Public Health Nursing." *American Journal of Public Health* 83 (1993): 1778–86.

_____. *No Place Like Home: A History of Nursing and Home Care in the United States.* Baltimore: Johns Hopkins University Press, 2001.

Bullough, Bonnie. "The Current Phase in the Development of Nurse Practice Acts." *St. Louis Law Journal* 28 (1985): 365–95.

Brush, Barbara, and Elizabeth A. Capezuti. "Revisiting a Nurse for All Settings: The Nurse Practitioner Movement, 1965–1995." *Journal of the American Academy of Nurse Practitioners* 8, 1 (January 1996): 5.

Calkin, Joy. "A Model for Advanced Nursing Practice." *Journal of Nursing Administration* 14, 1 (1984): 24–30.

Clinton, Catherine. *The Other Civil War: American Women in the Nineteenth Century.* 2nd ed. New York: Hill and Wang, 1999.

_____. *The Plantation Mistress: Woman's World in the Old South.* New York: Pantheon, 1982.

Crawley, Mildred. "Care of the Patient with Myocardial Infarction." *American Journal of Nursing* 61, 2 (February 1961): 68.

Christman, Luther. "Advanced Practice Nursing: Is the physician's assistant an accident of history or a failure to act? *Nursing Outlook* 46, 2 (1998): 56–59.

Daly, Barbara. *The Acute Care Nurse Practitioner.* New York: Springer Publishing Company, 1997.

Day, Hughes W. "History of Coronary Care Units." *American Journal of Cardiology* 30 (1972): 405.

_____. "An Intensive Coronary Care Area." *Diseases of the Chest* 44, 4 (1963): 424.

Diers, Donna. "Nurse-midwives and Nurse Anesthetists: The cutting edge in specialist practice." In L. H. Aiken and C. M. Fagin, eds., *Charting Nursing's Future: Agenda for the 1990s.* New York: J. B. Lippincott, 1991, 159–80.

Dock, Lavinia L. "An Experiment in Contagious Nursing." *American Journal of Nursing* 3 (1902–03): 927–33

_____. *Text-Book of Materia Medica for Nurses.* New York: G. P. Putnam's Sons, 1892.

_____. *Text-Book of Materia Medica for Nurses.* 7th ed. New York: G. P. Putnam's Sons, 1921.

Doyle, E., and J. Meurer. "Missouri Legislation and Litigation: Practicing medicine without a license." *Nurse Practitioner* 8 (1983): 41–44.

Draye, Mary Ann., and Marie A. Brown. "Surviving the Proving Ground: Lessons in Change from NP Pioneers." *The Nurse Practitioner* 25, 10 (2000): 60–71.

Drown, Lucy L. "A Successful Experiment." *American Journal of Nursing* 1 (July 1901): 729–31.

Duffus, R. L. *Lillian Wald, Neighbor and Crusader.* New York: Macmillan, 1938.

Duggar, Charlotte. "Letters from a Frontier Hospital." Reprint. *Quarterly Bulletin* 14, 4 (Spring 1940): 2.

Dye, Nancy. "Mary Breckenridge, The Frontier Nursing Service and the Introduction of Nurse-Midwifery in the United States." *The Bulletin of the History of Medicine* 57 (Winter 1983): 485–507.

Ettinger, Laura. "Nurse-Midwives, the Mass Media, and the Politics of Maternal Health Care in the United States, 1925–1955." *Nursing History Review* 7 (1999): 47–66.

Faddis, Margene O. "Eliminating Errors in Medication." *American Journal of Nursing* 39, 11 (November 1939): 1217–23.

_____. "New Drugs." *American Journal of Nursing* 41, 7 (July 1941): 759–63.

Ford, Loretta, and Henry Silver. "The Expanded Role of the Nurse in Child Care." *Nursing Outlook* 15, 8 (1967): 43–45.

Fairman, Julie. "Playing Doctor?: Nurse Practitioners, Physicians, and the Dilemma of Shared Practice." In *The Long Term View* [no eds.]. Andover, MA: Massachusetts School of Law at Andover, 1999, 27–35.

_____. "The Roots of Collaborative Practice: Nurse Practitioner Pioneers' Stories." *Nursing History Review* 10 (2002): 159–74

_____. "Watchful Vigilance: Nursing Care, Technology and the Development of Intensive Care Units." *Nursing Research* 41, 1 (January/February 1992): 56–60.

Fairman, Julie, and Joan E. Lynaugh. *Critical Care Nursing: A History.* Philadelphia: University of Pennsylvania Press, 1998.

Fantus, Bernard. *The Technic of Medication.* Chicago: Press of the American Medical Association, 1926.

Feudtner, Chris. *Bittersweet: Diabetes, Insulin and the Transformation of Illness.* Chapel Hill: University of North Carolina Press, 2003.

Foley, Edna. "Standing Orders." *American Journal of Nursing* 13 (March 1913): 451–53.

Ford, Loretta. "A Deviant Comes of Age." *Heart and Lung* 26, 2 (March–April, 1997): 87–91.

_____. "A Nurse for All Settings: The Nurse Practitioner." *Nursing Outlook* (August 1979): 516–20.

*Frank v. South*, 175, Ky. 416, 194, S.W. 375 (1917).

Frisbie, Charlotte J. *Navajo Medicine Bundles or Jish: Acquisition, Transmission and Disposition in the Past and Present.* Albuquerque: University of New Mexico Press, 1987.

Gill, Elizabeth. "Some Recent Developments in Drug Therapy." *American Journal of Nursing* 44, 8 (August 1944): 741–44.

Gilpin, Laura. *The Enduring Navaho.* Austin: University of Texas Press, 1974.

Geolot, Denise. "Federal Funding of Nurse Practitioner Education: Past Present and Future." *Nurse Practitioner Forum* 1, 3 (December 1990): 159–62.

Goodnow, Minnie. "Success in Teaching Materia Medica." *American Journal of Nursing* 7 (1906–1907): 703–704.

Grey, Michael R. *New Deal Medicine: The Rural Health Programs of the Farm Security Administration.* Baltimore: The Johns Hopkins University, 1999.

Hadley, Elizabeth H. "Nurse and Prescriptive Authority: A Legal and Economic Analysis." *American Journal of Law and Medicine,* 15, 2–3 (1989): 245–99.

Hamric, Ann B. "History and Overview of the CNS Role." In A. B. Hamric and Judith A. Spross, eds., *The Clinical Nurse Specialist in Theory and Practice.* 2nd ed. Philadelphia: W. B. Saunders, 1989, 3–18.

Harmer, B., and V. Henderson, eds. "Chapter 25: Administration of Medicines." In *Textbook of the Principles and Practice of Nursing.* 5th ed. New York: The MacMillan Co., 1955, 693–94.

Harris, Nancy, and Joan Hunziker-Dean. "Florence Henderson: The Art of Open–Drop Ether." *Nursing History Review* 9 (2001): 159–84.

Henderson, Florence. "The Nurse as Anesthetist." *American Journal of Nursing* (1909): 947–54.

Herb, Isabella C. "Accidents During and Following General Anesthesia." *Quarterly Supplement of Anesthesia and Analgesia, American Journal of Surgery* 30, 9 (1916): 297–302.

_____. "Administration of General Anesthetics with Special Reference to Ether and Chloroform." *Journal of the American Medical Association* 56 (1911): 1312–15.

Jacobson, Judith S. *The Greatest Good: A History of the John A. Hartford Foundation.* New York: John A. Hartford Foundation, 1984.

Jolly, E. *Nuns of the Battlefield.* Providence, RI: The Providence Visitor Press, 1927.

Jude, James R., William B. Kouwenhoven, and G. Guy Knickerbocker. "Cardiac Arrest." *JAMA* 178, 11 (December 16, 1961): 1063–70.

Jeans, Philip C., and Winifred Rand. *Essentials of Pediatrics for Nurses.* Philadelphia: J. B. Lippincott, 1938.

Hadley, Elizabeth H. "Nurses and Prescriptive Authority: A Legal and Economic Analysis." *American Journal of Law and Medicine* 15, 2–3 (1989): 245–99.

Hamilton, Diane. "The Cost of Caring: The Metropolitan Life Insurance Company's Visiting Nurse Service, 1909–1953." *Bulletin of the History of Medicine* 63, 3 (Fall 1989): 420.

Harper, Edwin. "Then and Now." *FNS Quarterly Bulletin* 64, 3 (1969): 6.

Herb, Isabella C. "Observations on One Thousand Consecutive Cases of Anesthesia in the Service of Dr. A. J. Ochsner, Augustana Hospital." *Chicago Medical Recorder* 15 (1898): 397–403.

Higby, Gregory. "Pharmacy in the American Century." *Pharmacy Times* 63 (1997): 16–24.

Hilts, Philip J. *Protecting America's Health: The FDA, Business, and One Hundred Years of Regulation.* New York: Knopf, 2003.

Hitchcock, Jane E. "Five Hundred Cases of Pneumonia." *American Journal of Nursing* 3 (1902–03): 169–75.

_____. "Methods of Nursing in Nurses' Settlement." *American Journal of Nursing* 7 (1906–07): 460–63.

Howell, Joel D. "Early Perceptions of the Electrocardiogram: from Arrhythmia to Infarction." *Bulletin of the History of Medicine* 58 (1984): 58.

Howell, Joel D. *Technology in the Hospital: Transforming Patient Care in the Early Twentieth Century.* Baltimore: Johns Hopkins University Press, 1996.

Hynson, H. P. "The Moral and Legal Responsibility of Nurses in the Purchase and Prescribing of Medicines." *American Journal of Nursing* 6 (1905–1906): 290–96.

Inglis, Antoinette, and Diane Kjervik. "Empowerment of Advanced Practice Nurse: Regulation Reform Needed to Increase Access to Care." *Journal of Law, Medicine and Ethics* 21, 2 (1993): 193–205.

Isquith, Robert. "Pediatric Nurse Practitioner Succeeds Mother as Indian Health Care Provider." *Commitment* 3, 3 (Summer 1978): 22–26.

Kalisch, Philip, and Bernice Kalisch. *The Advance of American Nursing.* 2nd ed. Boston: Little, Brown and Company, 1986.

Kassirer, Jerome. "What Role for Nurse Practitioners in Primary Care?" *The New England Journal of Medicine* 330, 3 (January 20, 1994): 204–205.

Keane, Ann, and Therese Richmond. "Tertiary Nurse Practitioners." *Image: Journal of Nursing Scholarship,* 25, 4 (1993): 281–84.

Keeling, Arlene, and Jeri Bigbee. "Chapter 1: The History of Advanced Practice Nursing in the United States." In *Advanced Nursing Practice: An Integrative Approach,* Ann Hamric, Judith Spross and Charlene Hanson, eds. Philadelphia: W. B. Saunders Co., 2005.

Kleinpell, Ruth. "Acute Care Nurse Practitioners: Roles and Practice Profiles." *American Association of Colleges of Nursing, Clinical Issues* 8, 1 (1997):156–62.

Koch, Larry, S. H. Pazaki, and James D. Campbell. "The First 20 Years of Nurse Practitioner Literature: An Evolution of Joint Practice Issues." *The Nurse Practitioner: A Journal of Primary Health Care* 17, 2 (February 1992): 62–71.

Kouwenhoven, William B., James R. Jude, and G. Guy Knickerbocker. "Closed Chest Cardiac Massage." *Journal of the American Medical Association* 173 (July 9, 1960): 1064–67.

Lambertson, Eleanor C. *Nursing Team Organization and Functioning.* New York: Bureau of Publications, Teachers College, Columbia University, 1953.

Lasby, Clarence G. *Eisenhower's Heart Attack.* Lawrence: University Press of Kansas, 1997.

Lawrence, Catherine S. *Sketch of Life and Labors of Miss Catherine S. Lawrence.* Albany, NY: James B. Lyon Publisher, 1896.

Leavitt, Judith. *Brought to Bed: Childbearing in America, 1750–1950.* Oxford: Oxford University Press, 1986.

Leavitt, Judith W. *Women and Health in America: Historical Readings.* 2nd ed. Madison: The University of Wisconsin Press, 1999.

Libster, Martha M. *Herbal Diplomats.* [No city]: Golden Apple Publications, 2004.

Lynaugh, Joan E., and Barbara L. Brush. *American Nursing: From Hospitals to Health Systems.* Cambridge and Oxford: Blackwell Publishers, Inc., 1996.

Lynaugh, Joan, Patricia Gerrity, and Gloria Hagopian. "Patterns of Practice: Master's Prepared Nurse Practitioners." *Journal of Nursing Education* 24, 7 (September 1985): 291–95.

Lytle, Albert T. "Materia Medica, Pharmacy and Therapeutics." *American Journal of Nursing* 6 (1905–1906): 217–24.

McAllister, William B. *Drug Diplomacy in the Twentieth Century: An International History.* London: Routledge, 2000.

Magaw, Alice. "Observations of 1092 Cases of Anesthesia from January 1, 1899 to January 1, 1900." *The St. Paul Medical Journal* 2 (May 1900): 306–311.

_____. "A Review of 14,000 Surgical Cases." *Bulletin of the American Association of Nurse Anesthetists* 7, 2 (May 1939): 66–68.

_____. "A Review of Over Fourteen Thousand Surgical Anesthesias." *Surgical Gynecology and Obstetrics* 3 (October 1906): 795–99.

Mahoney, Diane F. "Nurse Practitioners as Prescribers: Past Research Trends and Future Study Needs." *The Nurse Practitioner* 17, 1 (January 1992): 44–51.

Maher, Sister Mary D. *To Bind up the Wounds: Catholic Sister Nurses in the U.S. Civil War.* Baton Rouge: Louisiana State University Press, 2005.

McMechan, Hoeffer, MD, ed. "Editorial." *American Journal of Surgery, Anesthesia Supplement* 30 (July 1916): 90.

Mechanic, David, Lynn B. Rogut, and David C. Colby. *Policy Challenges in Modern Health Care.* Rutgers, NJ: Rutgers University Press, 2005.

Melosh, Barbara. *The Physician's Hand: Work Culture and Conflict in American Nursing.* Philadelphia: Temple University Press, 1982.

Meltzer, Lawrence E., Rose Pinneo, and J. Roderick Kitchell. *Intensive Coronary Care: A Manual for Nurses.* Rev. ed. Philadelphia: Charles Press, 1972.

Meriam, Lewis. *The Problem of Indian Administration.* Baltimore: The Johns Hopkins Press, 1928.

Metzger, Irvin D. "The Nurse as an Anesthetist." *Bulletin of the National Association of Nurse Anesthesia* 11, 3 (1936): 135–38.

Mitchell-DiCenso, A., G. Guyatt, M. Marrin, R. Goeree, A. Willan, et al. "A Controlled Trial of Nurse Practitioners in Neonatal Intensive Care." *Pediatrics,* 98, 6 (1996): 1143–48.

Montag, M. L., and M. Filson. "Administration of Medicines." *Nursing Arts.* Philadelphia: W. B. Saunders, Co., 1948, 482–87.

Mundinger, Mary O. "Twenty-first-century Primary Care: New Partnerships between Nurses and Doctors." *Academic Medicine* 77, 8 (August 2002): 776–80.

Nagle, E. Nora, RN. "The Mustard Pack." *American Journal of Nursing* 25, 6 (1925): 457–58.

National Organization of Nurse Practitioner Faculties (NONPF), *Criteria for*

*Evaluation of Nurse Practitioner Programs.* Washington, DC: National Task Force on Quality Nurse Practitioner Education, 1997.

Nightingale, Florence. *Notes on Nursing: What it is and What it is not. Commemorative Edition.* Philadelphia: J. B. Lippincot, 1992 (original publication, 1859).

Office of Technology Assessment, Nurse Practitioners, Physicians Assistants and Certified Nurse Midwives: A Policy Analysis (U.S. Congress, HCS 37, 1986).

Paul, George P. *A Textbook of Materia Medica for Nurses.* 6th ed. Philadelphia: W. B. Saunders, 1930.

Pinneo, Rose. "Machines in Perspective: Nursing in a Coronary Care Unit." *American Journal of Nursing* 65 (1965): 76–79.

Pitts Mosley, Marie O. "Satisfied to Carry the Bag: Three Black Community Health Nurses' Contributions to Health Care Reform, 1900–1937." *Nursing History Review* 4 (1996): 65–82.

Pougiales, Jean. "The First Anesthetizers at the Mayo Clinic." *Journal of the American Association of Nurse Anesthetists* 38, no. 3 (June 1970): 235–41.

Rand, Winefred. "Impression of a Public Health Nursing Service in the Kentucky Mountains." *American Journal of Nursing* 29, 5 (May 1929): 527–30.

Reverby, Susan. *Ordered to Care: The Dilemma of American Nursing, 1850–1945.* New York: Cambridge University Press, 1987.

Rinker, Sylvia. "To Cultivate a Feeling of Confidence: The Nursing of Obstetric Patients, 1890–1940." *Nursing History Review* 8 (2000): 117–142.

_____. "The Real Challenge: Lessons from Obstetric Nursing History." *Journal of Obstetric, Gynecologic, and Neonatal Nursing* 29, 1 (2000): 100–106.

Rogers, Lina L. "A Year's Work for the Children in New York Schools." *American Journal of Nursing* 4 (1906): 181–84.

_____. "The Nurse in the Public School." *American Journal of Nursing* 5 (1905): 764–73.

_____. "School Nursing in New York City." *American Journal of Nursing* 3 (1903): 448–50.

_____. "Some Phases of School Nursing." *American Journal of Nursing* 8 (1908): 966.

Rogers, Martha E. "Nursing: to be or not to be." *Nursing Outlook* 20 (1972): 42–46.

Rooks, Judith. *Midwifery and Childbirth in America.* Philadelphia: Temple University Press, 1997.

Rosenberg, Charles E. "Social Class and Medical Care in 19th–Century America: The Rise and Fall of the Dispensary." *Journal of the History of Medicine and Allied Sciences* 29 (1974): 32–54.

Rude, Anna. "The Sheppard-Towner Act in Relation to Public Health." *Journal of the American Medical Association* 20, 12 (September 16, 1922): 959–64.

Ruffing-Rahal, Mary Ann. "The Navajo Experience of Elizabeth Forster, Public Health Nurse." *Nursing History Review* 3 (1995): 173–88.

Safriet, Barbara J. "Health Care Dollars and Regulatory Sense: the Role of Advance Practice Nursing." *Yale Journal on Regulation,* 9, 2 (Summer 1992): 417–88.

Sandelowski, Margarete. "The Physician's Eyes: American Nursing and the Diagnostic Revolution in Medicine." *Nursing History Review* 8 (2000): 3–38.

Sandweiss, Martha A. *Denizens of the Desert: A Tale in Word and Picture of Life among the Navajo Indians.* Albuquerque: University of New Mexico Press, 1988.

Sarnecky, Mary T. *A History of the U.S. Army Nurse Corps.* Philadelphia: University of Pennsylvania Press, 1999.

Shah, H., K. Brutlomesso, D. Sullivan, and J. Lattanzio. "An Evaluation of the Role and Practices of the Acute Care Nurse Practitioner." *AACN Clinical Issues* 8, 1 (1997): 147–55.

Smith, Susan L. "White Nurses, Black Midwives, and Public Health in Mississippi, 1920–1950." *Nursing History Review* 2 (1994): 29–49.

[na]. "Some Specialists: Mary Breckenridge, RN, Nurse-Midwife." *American Journal of Nursing* 30, 3 (March 1930): 311–314.

Stein, Leonard. "The Doctor-Nurse Game." *Archives of General Psychiatry* 16 (1967): 699–703.

Stevens, Rosemary. *American Medicine and the Public Interest.* Berkeley: University of California Press, 1998.

Stevens, Rosemary. *In Sickness and in Wealth, American Hospitals in the Twentieth Century.* New York: Basic Books, 1989.

Strickland, Robert. "Isabella Coler Herb, MD: An early leader in anesthesiology." *Anesthesia and Analgesia* 80, 3 (March 1995): 600–605.

Summers, Vanda. "Saddle-bag and Log Cabin Technic." *American Journal of Nursing* 38, 11 (1938): 1183–84.

Taussig, Frederick J. "The Nurse-Midwife." *Public Health Nursing Quarterly* 6 (1914): 33–39.

*A Tenement Story: The History of 97 Orchard Street and the Lower East Side Tenement Museum.* New York: The Lower East Side Tenement Museum, 2004.

Thatcher, Virginia S. *History of Anesthesia with Emphasis on the Nurse Specialist.* Philadelphia: Lippincott, 1953.

Tirpak, Helen. "The Frontier Nursing Service: Fifty years in the Mountains." *Nursing Outlook* 23, 5 (May 1975): 308–310.

Trennert, Robert. *White Man's Medicine: Government Doctors and the Navajo, 1863–1955.* Albuquerque: University of New Mexico Press, 1998.

Truckey, Frances. "Anesthesia and Anesthetics." *The American Journal of Nursing* 11 (1911): 803–806.

United States Public Health Service (USPHS). *Contagious and Infectious Diseases among the Indians.* Senate Document #1083, 62nd Congress, 3rd Session. Washington, DC: Government Printing Office, 1913, 1–85.

Wald, Lillian. *House on Henry Street.* New York: H. Holt and Company, 1915.

_____. "The Nurses' Settlement." Official Reports of Societies, *American Journal of Nursing* 2 (1901–02): 386–87

_____. "The Nurses' Settlement in New York." *American Journal of Nursing* 2, 8 (May 1902): 567–73

_____. "The Treatment of Families in Which There Is Sickness." *American Journal of Nursing* 4 (1904): 13.

Wall, Barbra Mann. *Unlikely Entrepreneurs: Catholic Sisters and the Hospital Marketplace, 1865–1925.* Columbus: The Ohio State University Press, 2005.

Weeks-Shaw, Clara. *Textbook of Nursing.* New York: D. Appleton and Company, 1902.

Whelan, Jean. "Smaller and Cheaper: The Chicago Hourly Nursing Service, 1926–1957." *Nursing History Review* 10 (2002): 83–108.

Wile, Ira S. "The Relation of the Public Health Nurse to the Practicing Physicians: The Viewpoint of the Physician." *American Journal of Public Health* (1924): 106–11.

Willeford, Mary B. *Income and Health in Remote Rural Areas: A Study of 400 Families in Leslie County Kentucky.* New York City: FNS Inc., 1932.

## Women, Gender, and Health
### Susan L. Smith and Nancy Tomes, Series Editors

This series focuses on the history of women and health, but also includes studies that address gender and masculinity. Works in the series examine the history of sickness, health, and healing in relation to health workers, activists, and patients. They also explore the ways in which issues of gender, race, ethnicity, and health have reflected and shaped beliefs, values, and power dynamics in society.

*A Social History of Wet Nursing: From Breast to Bottle*
Janet Golden

*And Sin No More: Social Policy and Unwed Mothers in Cleveland, 1855–1990*
Marian J. Morton

*Any Friend of the Movement: Networking for Birth Control, 1920–1940*
Jimmy Elaine Wilkinson Meyer

*Beyond the Reproductive Body: The Politics of Women's Health and Work in Early Victorian England*
Marjorie Levine-Clark

*Bodies of Technology: Women's Involvement with Reproductive Medicine*
Edited by Ann R. Saetnan, Nelly Oudshoorn, and Marta Kirejczyk

*Crack Mothers: Pregnancy, Drugs, and the Media*
Drew Humphries

*Don't Kill Your Baby: Public Health and the Decline of Breastfeeding in the Nineteenth and Twentieth Centuries*
Jacqueline H. Wolf

*Dying to Be Beautiful: The Fight for Safe Cosmetics*
Gwen Kay

*Handling the Sick: The Women of St. Luke's and the Nature of Nursing, 1892–1937*
Tom Olson and Eileen Walsh

*Listen to Me Good: The Story of an Alabama Midwife*
Margaret Charles Smith and Linda Janet Holmes